Healing with Apple Cider Vinegar

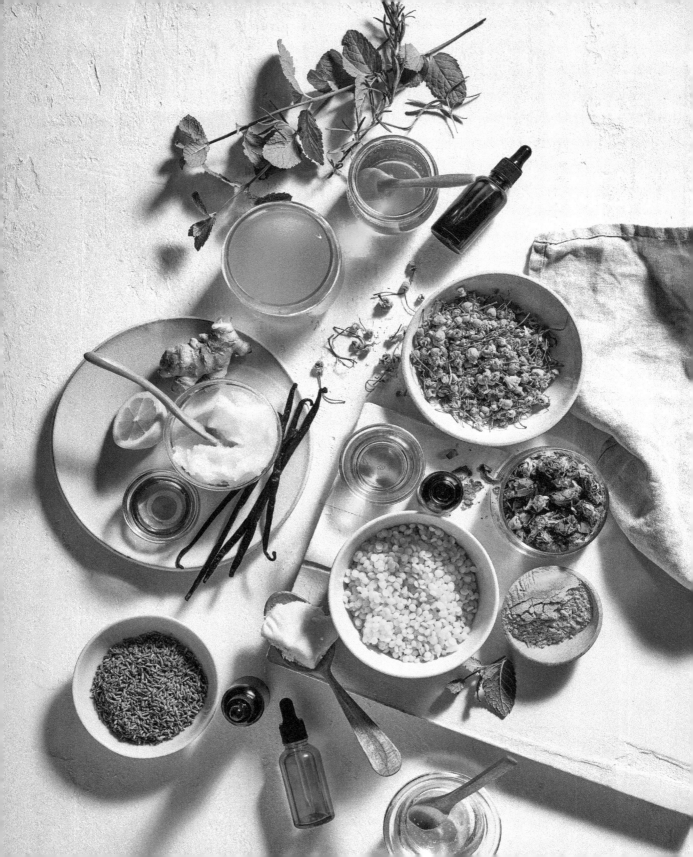

Healing with
Apple Cider Vinegar

115 Recipes for Health,
Beauty, and Home

KAYLEIGH CHRISTINA CLARK

ROCKRIDGE
PRESS

Interior and Cover Designer: Lisa Forde
Art Producer: Sue Bischofberger
Editor: Shannon Criss
Production Manager: Giraud Lorber
Production Editor: Matt Burnett

Photography: © 2019 Emulsion Studio, cover and pp. ii, vi, ix, 14, 64, and 112; © Helene Dujardin, p. xii; © Madeleine Steinbach/shutterstock, p. 143.

Author photo: © Hannah Claire Photography.

ISBN: Print 978-1-64152-852-8 | Ebook 978-1-64152-853-5

RO

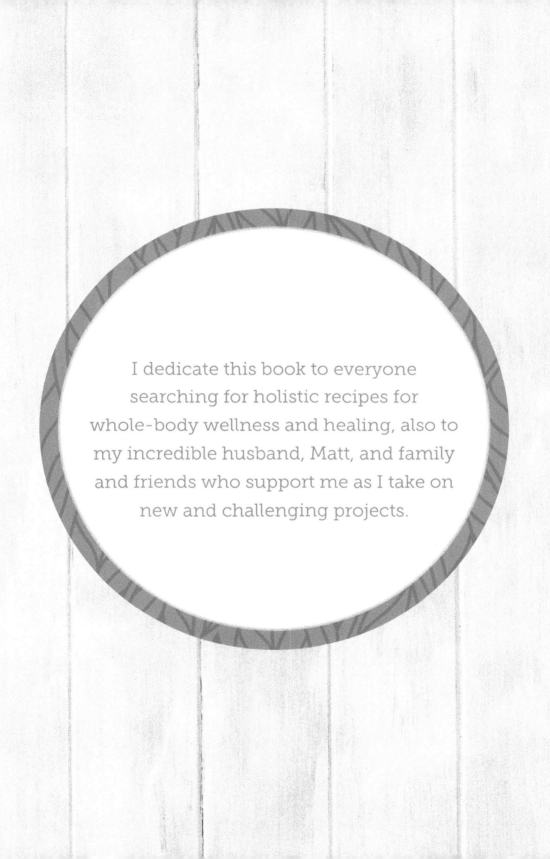

I dedicate this book to everyone searching for holistic recipes for whole-body wellness and healing, also to my incredible husband, Matt, and family and friends who support me as I take on new and challenging projects.

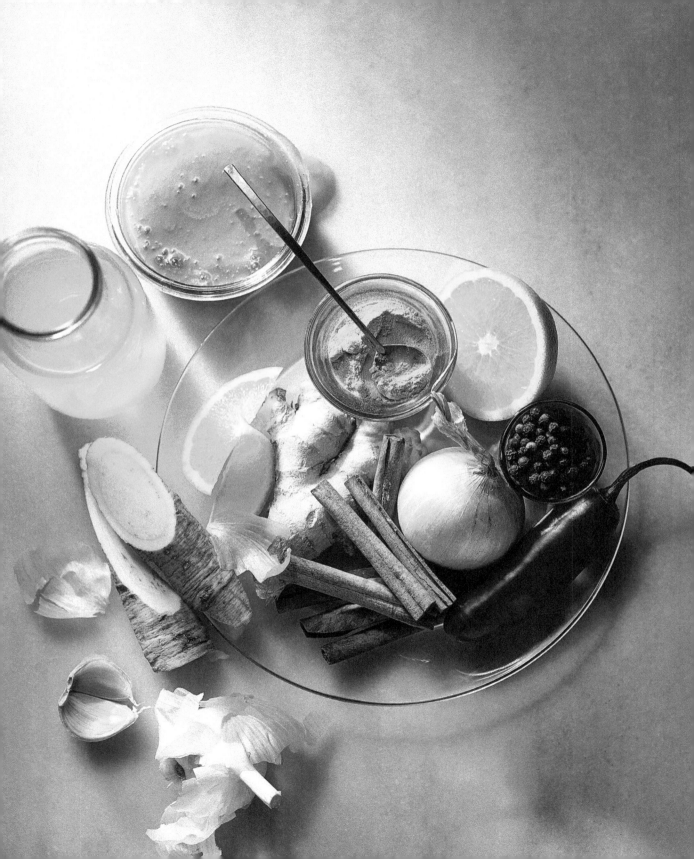

Contents

Introduction

Taking a holistic approach to wellness can change your life. I know this is true because I have experienced it firsthand. As a certified holistic health and wellness coach, nutritionist, and cofounder of CLEARstem Skincare, I now take a very natural approach to life and exude enthusiasm and positivity. Life was not always this way for me, so before you turn the page, know that you are not alone.

During my adolescence, I suffered from chronic migraines, viral infections, allergies, acne, and anxiety. I remember leaving school so many times feeling ill or experiencing the heart-pounding, debilitating feeling of anxiety that made me sick to my stomach. Every time this happened, my doctor prescribed yet another medication to help with my symptoms. When I got older, I got sick in a different way. I started to become allergic to many things, suffered from severe cystic acne, and experienced sudden rapid weight loss. I was chronically stressed, and I developed ulcers on my uterus, as well as a breast tumor.

One day a friend suggested I see a naturopathic doctor. That experience changed my life. I was introduced to a new way of thinking about and approaching health. I also learned that I was suffering from leaky gut, a hyperactive liver, and celiac disease, which is an autoimmune response to eating gluten. My body was attacking itself, and on top of that, I had been experiencing major inflammation.

To begin healing, I was instructed to remove all gluten, dairy, processed foods, and other inflammatory foods from my diet. For the first time, I started to feel better, and over time, I felt crazy good.

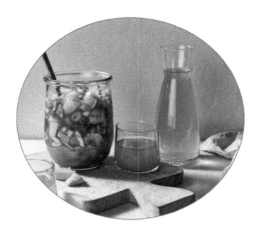

I made a lot of other changes in my life to increase healing. One of those changes was introducing apple cider vinegar into my lifestyle. My doctor had suggested I start including it in my morning routine to boost stomach acid production. Because I was having so many digestive issues, my stomach was drastically low in acid, making it difficult for my body to digest food properly. The very first thing I started making was my Morning Digestion Tonic (page 48). After I removed all caffeine from my diet, this tonic became my new go-to morning beverage.

Over time I fell in love with apple cider vinegar's versatility. In addition to its healing benefits, it also has a place in beauty regimens and can be used as a base for dozens of nontoxic cleaners and disinfectants. Throughout this book I share my many uses for apple cider vinegar. I have written recipes to aid digestion and gut health, and remedies for common ailments such as anxiety and joint pain; beauty regimens for acne, hyperpigmentation, and dry or oily hair; and mixtures for use around the home.

My own healing journey lit a fire within me to help others. I am on a mission to educate and inspire people to find their own healing journeys through a holistic approach to wellness.

Part I

Understanding the Healing Properties of Apple Cider Vinegar

The goal of this book is to improve health and wellness and set a path to looking and feeling your best through the use of apple cider vinegar. Before we jump into the recipes and remedies, it is worthwhile to learn about the amazing benefits of apple cider vinegar and why it works so well for a variety of uses. Chapter 1 will explain its benefits, recount its history, describe how to use it safely, and answer frequently asked questions. I hope understanding what apple cider vinegar is and how it works will inspire you to incorporate it into your life.

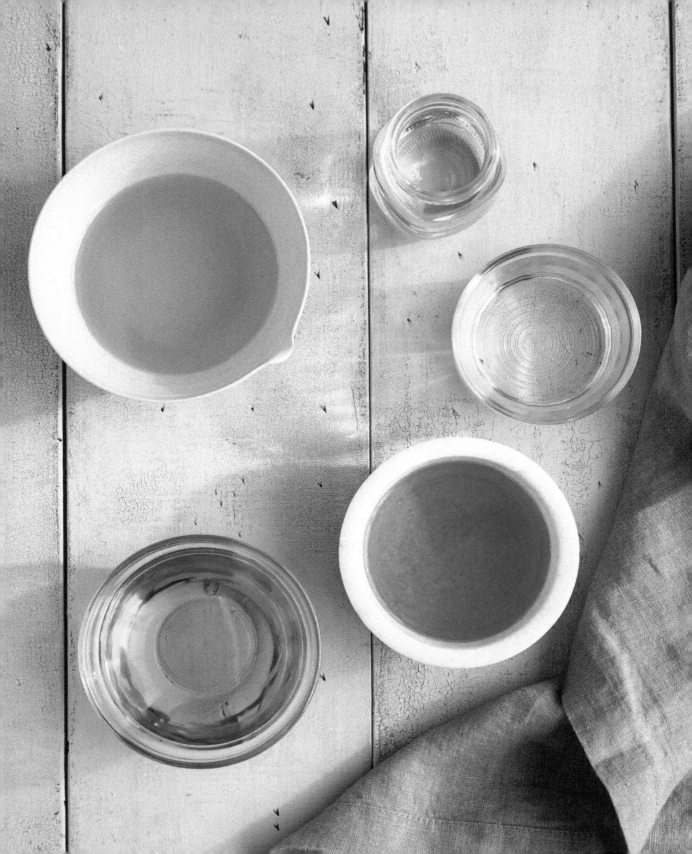

The Basics

Apple cider vinegar is not a miracle cure. Just like any supplement you introduce into your diet, it is meant to enhance an already balanced diet. Think of apple cider vinegar as your new sidekick. When you incorporate it with whole foods, you are on the road to sustainable long-term health. Incorporating apple cider vinegar into both my diet and lifestyle has been an absolute game changer!

What Is Apple Cider Vinegar?

Apple cider vinegar is a vinegar made from apples that have been crushed, distilled, and fermented to form healthy probiotics, enzymes, and high levels of acetic acid. It has been used for thousands of years for household and cooking purposes and is best known for its healing properties.

The Benefits of Apple Cider Vinegar

With uses of apple cider vinegar including boosting weight loss, supporting digestion and gut health, improving insulin function, and lowering cholesterol, you'll learn the importance of incorporating apple cider vinegar into your daily life and why it should be a staple in your kitchen, bathroom, and medicine cabinet. If you are just starting to experiment with apple cider vinegar, you may question the validity of its benefits. Let's take a look.

IT HELPS WITH DIGESTION

I have had many clients incorporate apple cider vinegar into their diets and notice a major improvement in their digestion, including issues with acid reflux. A key component of healthy digestion is the presence of enough stomach acid to break down food. Low stomach acid leads to bacteria buildup, gas, and bloating: everything we don't want! Apple cider vinegar helps increase stomach acid levels, which in turn helps you correctly digest food. It also prevents backflow into the esophagus, reducing both acid reflux and heartburn.

IT HELPS BOOST YOUR IMMUNE SYSTEM

For centuries, apple cider vinegar has been used to ward off common illnesses. I suffer from seasonal allergies, and this natural product has been my go-to home remedy. Its wealth of healing properties is due to the fact that it contains many antimicrobials and antiseptic properties, as well as vitamins, minerals, and enzymes that help boost your body's own natural ability to heal itself. Most germs cannot survive in the acidic environment apple cider vinegar creates, making it the perfect addition to your diet when you are feeling sick.

IT HELPS WITH WEIGHT LOSS

Studies have shown that the acetic acid found in apple cider vinegar helps suppress your appetite. This benefit can be especially useful if you love to snack between meals. Incorporating apple cider vinegar is my number one tip for my clients who struggle with the constant urge to snack. Apple cider vinegar can also help reduce bloating, increase your metabolism, and give you an energy boost. However, don't think that apple cider vinegar will make weight just fall off. I always recommend it be used as a supplement to a healthy, balanced diet.

IT HELPS WITH DIABETES

Many people with type 2 diabetes have experienced the positive effects of apple cider vinegar, specifically with keeping their blood sugar levels balanced, a claim that research has supported. A study in *Diabetes Journal* observed that people with type 2 diabetes who weren't taking insulin but took two tablespoons of apple cider vinegar before bed had lower glucose levels in the morning. Another study in *Diabetes Care* showed that consuming apple cider vinegar improved insulin sensitivity by up to 34 percent in those with either insulin resistance or type 2 diabetes.

IT PROMOTES HEALTHY SKIN, HAIR, AND NAILS

Apple cider vinegar is a simple way to give your beauty routine a boost. It can help treat acne, dandruff, and sunburn, as well as remove buildup on your scalp to give you soft, shiny hair. Because it contains acetic acid and lactic acid, apple cider vinegar has been shown to inhibit the growth of the bacteria responsible for causing acne. It has also been known to improve the texture and pigmentation of skin and strengthen nails to promote growth.

IT IS A GREAT HOUSEHOLD REMEDY

In addition to its positive health and beauty effects, apple cider vinegar is a great addition to your cleaning supplies. It is an ingredient in dozens of household remedies for cleaning, disinfecting, killing insects, and even helping your garden flourish.

Homemade Apple Cider Vinegar

Like alcohol, apple cider vinegar is made in a two-step fermentation process. In fact, the French translation of vinegar is "sour wine." Though there are several ways to make apple cider vinegar, the most common is by combining apples, water, sugar—and time.

STEP 1: When you fully submerge apples in a mixture of sugar and water without any exposure to oxygen, the apples begin to ferment. In the fermentation process, the yeast naturally occurring in the fruit transforms the liquid into alcohol. This process typically takes a few weeks. After that, the second step can begin.

STEP 2: The alcohol is exposed to bacteria, turning it into acetic acid, which is the active component of apple cider vinegar. The entire process can take anywhere from a few weeks to months. When the final product is ready, there is no alcohol left, only acetic acid.

THE MOTHER: When apple cider vinegar ferments naturally, a grouping of bacteria and yeast forms, which is known as the "mother." Containing both healthy bacteria and enzymes, the mother is what gives apple cider vinegar its plethora of health benefits. The bacteria in the mother are commonly known as probiotics. Probiotics are great for your immune system, digestive system, and mental health. The enzymes found in the mother support your digestive system by helping your body break down foods. Many health advocates believe that you are getting the maximum benefits of apple cider vinegar only if the mother is left in. You can easily spot the mother by seeing if your apple cider vinegar has murky substances floating around inside. Don't worry—this is a good thing!

Whether apple cider vinegar is being consumed internally for health benefits or used topically, you will want to buy **ORGANIC, RAW,** and **UNFILTERED.** This means that nothing was added, no pesticides were used on the apples, and it wasn't artificially processed. You will also want to make sure that the mother is in the apple cider vinegar you are purchasing because it contains the majority of the benefits.

The History of Apple Cider Vinegar

It may seem like apple cider vinegar came out of nowhere to become a hot health trend. In recent years, breakthrough research has been released regarding the benefits to gut and digestive health from the ingestion of probiotics. With apple cider vinegar's wealth of probiotics and its easy accessibility, it was only a matter of time before it became a trendy item to have in your pantry. It has an array of purposes, but it is not new. Believe it or not, apple cider vinegar has been used for thousands of years for health, beauty, and home purposes.

IN HEALTH

The practice of fermentation dates to 5000 BCE, when the Babylonians made wine from date palms. Over time, the practice progressed to making apple cider from apples, and then the Greeks and Romans began making apple cider vinegar as a by-product of their apple cider. When it was discovered that vinegar had healing properties, physicians began prescribing it to treat and prevent illnesses. Hippocrates, who is known as "the father of medicine," prescribed it to treat wounds, sores, and other ailments. Throughout history it has been used for its detoxifying, cleansing, and energizing properties. Just as you may see coconuts sold at street markets today, apple cider vinegar was once sold on the streets as an energizing beverage, giving strength and power. During the American Civil War and World War I, its antiseptic and antibacterial properties were recognized, and it was used to treat wounds on the battlefield. Progressing to modern times, apple cider vinegar is a well-known remedy in the world of health and is recommended by many US medical practitioners. Internally, the consumption of apple cider vinegar has been known to help with losing weight, reducing cholesterol, lowering blood sugar levels, fighting diabetes, improving digestion, cleaning wounds, and more.

IN BEAUTY

As you scroll through the Internet or walk through the beauty aisle, you will find that apple cider vinegar is used in a variety of skin products and remedies. Using apple cider vinegar for beauty is an ancient practice that has existed since the Roman Empire. The best-known historical use of apple cider vinegar is believed to have been practiced by Cleopatra, who was known for her intoxicating beauty; it is said that she used it to cleanse and tone her face. Apple cider vinegar contains high acid levels that aid in balancing the skin's pH levels, making it helpful for controlling oily or dry skin, lightening pigmentation, reducing acne, and removing dirt buildup. It is also beneficial for killing bacteria and calming itchy, irritated skin, providing relief from eczema, sunburn, and other skin irritations. Apple cider vinegar also helps remove product buildup in the hair, leaving you with clean, shiny, silky-feeling hair.

IN THE HOME

One of the first uses of vinegar was by the Babylonians to preserve food and as a condiment. This use dates as far back as 5000 BCE. Apple cider vinegar is a staple in many pantries and has been used for many purposes in the home because of its antibacterial, antiseptic, and cleansing properties. It is a safe, inexpensive option to use around the house rather than turning to harsh chemical cleaners. Apple cider vinegar works to kill bacteria on surfaces while effectively removing surface dirt and excess buildup, and it is easily added to mixtures for various cleaning and disinfecting uses. You can find it in a variety of recipes to help remove grease, deodorize clothes and rags, remove stains, unclog drains, remove mildew, and more.

Precautions

When you introduce anything new into your diet, awareness of quantity and usage is very important. There is a wide array of healthy foods that, when consumed in excess, can have negative effects. If you are not used to consuming apple cider vinegar daily, it is important to note that you should practice safe use regarding quantity and frequency in the beginning.

SUGGESTED CONCENTRATION

Apple cider vinegar is an acid, and acids can burn, so you must dilute it before consuming it. The suggested dilution is one to two tablespoons of apple cider vinegar per eight ounces of liquid. This will ensure that your esophagus lining is not compromised. Another precaution is to consume apple cider vinegar through a straw to protect your tooth enamel. Perhaps consider investing in a reusable straw.

When using apple cider vinegar topically, it is important to avoid applying pure vinegar directly to your skin. I always recommend a patch test first. To do this test, dilute one tablespoon of apple cider vinegar in four ounces of water, mix, and apply on a small part of your skin. The inside of your wrist is a perfect place to start. If you do not have any adverse reactions, you can move forward with using apple cider vinegar as a remedy on the skin.

 I recommend apple cider vinegar to almost all of my clients, especially those who struggle with digestive issues. Apple cider vinegar diluted in water is a great way to naturally increase stomach acid levels to aid in the digestive process, to prevent heartburn, and to provide your gut with a healthy dose of beneficial bacteria. I love having my clients start the day with a warm cup of water with some apple cider vinegar and lemon juice to get their digestive juices flowing straight off the bat, and clients see huge improvements with this! Apple cider vinegar is also great for appetite regulation and balancing blood sugar, which is why so many of my clients benefit from using it regularly. Even though I love apple cider vinegar, there are dangers of overusing it or using it incorrectly. Undiluted apple cider vinegar can be way too acidic for the skin and/or digestive tract, causing major irritation. It is also important to use a straw when consuming it, because apple cider vinegar can contribute to the erosion of tooth enamel. As long as clients are diluting the ACV, they usually have no problems, but there is a subset of people who actually experience more digestive issues and/or hypoglycemia from consuming apple cider vinegar. It is always important to be aware of how something affects your body specifically, and honor that."

—**CHRISTINA RICE,** Nutritional Therapy Practitioner, Primal Health Coach, and Reiki Practitioner

CAUTIONS FOR OVERUSE

Although it is easy to get caught up in all the benefits of apple cider vinegar, know that it is possible to have too much of a good thing. When trying out all these recipes, be aware of overusing apple cider vinegar. When consumed in excess, it can actually have negative effects on the digestive system, causing distress and irritation rather than promoting benefits. Something else to be aware of is the effect it has on oral health. Anything acidic, such as soft drinks, fruit juices, and yes, vinegar, have been shown to damage tooth enamel and burn the esophagus. So be sure to consume minimally and avoid excess; you can refer to the FAQ section (page 10) for more information regarding this caution.

 While there are a wide variety of benefits to apple cider vinegar, I would still encourage precautions to prevent damage to teeth, in particular to the enamel. Apple cider vinegar is an acidic substance that can lead to breakdown of enamel if it is in contact with the teeth for an extended amount of time. This breakdown can lead to an increased risk of cavity formation. An easy way to prevent that contact is to use a straw while drinking the vinegar, or to simply rinse your mouth with water after drinking the vinegar to clean the teeth of the acid."

—**SEENA GHETMIRI,** Dentist

Materials Needed

As you prepare the recipes in this book you will need some simple kitchen items that you likely already have on hand, such as pots and pans, bowls, spoons, measuring cups, and glasses. The following items are some you may not already own and will want to have to make your storage easier.

» **GLASS DROPPER BOTTLES:** Amazon has the widest selection of these in a variety of sizes. You can also purchase them in bulk for multiple recipes or if you are making any of these recipes as gifts.

» **MASON JARS:** These come in a variety of sizes—from smaller ones in the beauty section to larger quart sizes in the health section—and are wonderful for storage. Please check the recipe for recommended storage before you begin, as well as recipe yield to inform the jar size.

» **GLASS SPRAY BOTTLES:** For purchasing online, I have found Amazon has the most options. If you want to shop in a store, most Walmart stores also carry these. I recommend using glass mainly because it is environmentally friendly. If you prefer plastic, or if that is the easiest option, feel free to use it.

Frequently Asked Questions

After reading all this information about apple cider vinegar, you may still have a few more questions. I know that before incorporating anything new into my diet, I sure do. These are some of the queries I have received from my clients, as well as general questions that have been posted on social media when I share my apple cider vinegar routines.

Q: *How much apple cider vinegar can be consumed daily?*

A: You may receive conflicting advice regarding this question. However, there are currently no scientific studies that have been published on the optimal dosage of apple cider vinegar. I believe in listening to your body and doing everything in moderation. With that said, I would avoid consuming more than four tablespoons a day, and those doses should be spread over at least a six- to eight-hour period. For example, you might make a morning beverage with apple cider vinegar and then also have an evening beverage that includes it. If you are feeling great with that amount, awesome! If you notice any adverse reactions, dial back to one to two tablespoons total per day and see how you feel.

Q: *Is apple cider vinegar a probiotic?*

A: This requires a two-part answer. The first part is no; apple cider vinegar itself is not a probiotic. What it does contain is pectin, which encourages the growth of good bacteria that is beneficial for digestion. The second part is that the mother in unfiltered apple cider vinegar does contain healthy bacteria, also known as probiotics. If you want those probiotics in your apple cider vinegar, make sure you are buying it raw, organic, and unfiltered.

Q: *Is apple cider vinegar considered a superfood?*

A: Apple cider vinegar is packed with naturally occurring nutrients, including acetic acid, alpha hydroxy acid, calcium, iron, magnesium, pectin, and potassium. When you have apple cider vinegar that also includes the mother, you are adding healthy bacteria and enzymes. With all these nutrients come the benefits for gut health, digestive health, mental health, and whole-body wellness. This makes apple cider vinegar, without a doubt, a superfood.

Q: *Does it matter if I purchase organic apple cider vinegar?*

A: If you are using apple cider vinegar strictly for cleaning purposes, such as removing stains and mildew, cleaning surfaces, and freshening rags and sponges, buying organic is not as important because you are using it only for its antibacterial and antiseptic properties. However, I do recommend buying it raw and unfiltered because highly processed apple cider vinegar is heated to a high temperature, which kills the properties that work best for cleaning. When purchasing apple cider vinegar for consumption and topical use, I always recommend buying organic. Apples are on the Dirty Dozen list published annually by the Environmental Working Group (EWG). This list includes the fruits and vegetables that have the highest amount of pesticides when grown conventionally rather than organically. If pesticides exist on the apples, and the apples are used to make the vinegar, you are also consuming those chemicals.

Q: *When is the best time to consume apple cider vinegar?*

A: Apple cider vinegar is best taken on an empty stomach before eating. This will maximize your body's ability to digest food, and it will also increase the health benefits. It is important to note that you should not consume apple cider vinegar immediately after eating because it can delay digestion, causing an interruption in the way your body processes your meal.

Part II

Nature's Prescriptions

N ow that you have read about the healing properties of apple cider vinegar, it is time to dive into the recipes. The following chapters offer a wealth of ways to incorporate apple cider vinegar into all aspects of your life. Chapter 2 focuses on recipes relating to health, chapter 3 outlines applications for beauty, and chapter 4 will help you keep your home fresh and clean.

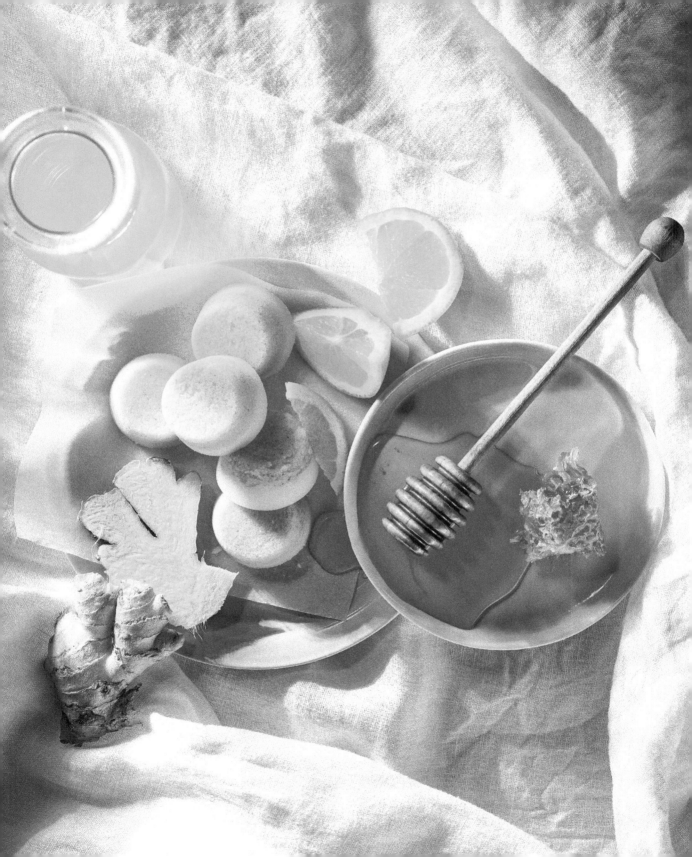

CHAPTER 2

Health

O ne of the oldest uses of apple cider vinegar is medicinal. In this chapter, we showcase its health role. Here you will find dozens of recipes for a variety of internal and external ailments. Internally, we cover illnesses and disorders such as acid reflux, poor digestion, cold and flu, migraines, and bloating. Externally, we cover health concerns such as insect bites, cuts and scrapes, and cramping.

Prevention and Wellness

This section addresses a wide variety of common ailments, including recipes for colds, sore throats, insect bites, relaxation, and boosting energy.

FEATURED RECIPES: Cold-Buster Shot (16), Sore Throat Buster (17), Peppermint Throat Gargle (18), Fire Cider Tonic (19), Eucalyptus Sinus Cleanser (20), Bone Broth Latte (21), Immunity-Boosting Golden Latte (22), Deep Sleep Spray (23), Blueberry-Lavender Stress-Reducing Smoothie (24), Unwind and Relax Reishi Elixir (25), Mood-Boosting Mocktail (26), Energizing Cordyceps Latte (27), Afternoon Pick-Me-Up Tonic (28), Liver Detox Elixir (29), Simple Insect Repellent (30), Lavender Afterbite Treatment (31), and Bee Sting Treatment (32).

ORANGE-GINGER CONSTIPATION BITES, PAGE 51

COLD-BUSTER SHOT

YIELD: 3 CUPS, OR 12 (2-OUNCE) SERVINGS | PREP TIME: 5 MINUTES

RECOMMENDED STORAGE: Store in a large, sealed glass jar in the refrigerator for up to 1 week.

Orange and lemon juices are high in vitamin C and antioxidants, giving your body the vitamins and nutrients it needs to fight off infection. Ginger helps soothe a sore throat and kills off rhinoviruses, which are known to be the cause of some forms of the common cold. Both turmeric and cayenne pepper are spices that are known natural remedies for preventing colds, and they help clear out sinus passages. Oil of oregano is a powerful antimicrobial and antioxidant that supports the immune system and fights against infectious bacteria. It is known as "nature's antibiotic."

1 orange, peeled

1 lemon, peeled

2 inches ginger root, peeled and roughly chopped

2 cups water

4 tablespoons apple cider vinegar

1 tablespoon turmeric

¼ teaspoon cayenne pepper

20 drops oil of oregano

1. In a blender, process the peeled orange, lemon, and ginger.

2. Pour the mixture into a glass jar and add the water, apple cider vinegar, turmeric, cayenne pepper, and oil of oregano. Cover and shake well to combine.

3. Shake well before each use. Consume one 2-ounce shot every morning and afternoon.

SORE THROAT BUSTER

YIELD: 8 OUNCES | PREP TIME: 10 MINUTES | INFUSION TIME: 1 HOUR

RECOMMENDED STORAGE: Store in a glass spray bottle in the refrigerator for up to 1 year.

This throat spray will provide immediate relief to a sore throat and help your body defend against illness. Studies have shown that echinacea helps fight infection by increasing the number of white blood cells in your body. It can also help shorten the length of a cold and accelerate your body's healing. Peppermint has anti-inflammatory effects and will provide relief to an aggravated throat, and raw honey can serve as a natural cough suppressant by coating mucous membranes. The combination of these ingredients will ease the irritation of a sore throat, suppress coughing, and help speed the healing process.

3 tablespoons dried echinacea

3 tablespoons dried peppermint leaves

Dash cayenne pepper

¾ cup boiling water

¼ cup apple cider vinegar

2 teaspoons raw honey

1. To make the herbal water, put the echinacea, peppermint, and cayenne pepper in a mug and pour the boiling water over the mixture.

2. Let the herbs infuse for at least 1 hour and then strain them out.

3. In a glass spray bottle, combine the herbal water, apple cider vinegar, and honey. Cover and shake well to combine.

4. Shake the bottle well before each use and spray a few pumps directly on the back of your throat.

PEPPERMINT THROAT GARGLE

YIELD: 1 (6-OUNCE) SERVING | PREP TIME: 10 MINUTES | COOK TIME: 2 MINUTES

RECOMMENDED STORAGE: Storage is not recommended.

This throat gargle will ease a dry cough, loosen phlegm, and help reduce throat pain. Apple cider vinegar kills bacteria and eases irritation by loosening phlegm. Salt relieves infections by drawing fluids from your mouth and throat, breaks up the mucus, and reduces irritation. Peppermint works to thin the mucus in your throat and serves as a decongestant. When you combine these ingredients, the result provides a major weapon for fighting inflammation in your throat.

½ cup water

¼ cup apple cider vinegar

1 teaspoon salt

2 to 3 drops peppermint essential oil

1. Heat the water in a pot over low heat until it is warm but not hot.

2. Pour the warm water into a cup and add the apple cider vinegar, salt, and peppermint essential oil.

3. Mix with a spoon until the salt is completely dissolved.

4. Take a large sip of the salt-water mixture and gargle for 30 seconds. Swish the water around your mouth, then spit it out.

5. Repeat the last step until all the water is gone.

USAGE TIP: Use this remedy 3 to 4 times a day until your throat is no longer sore.

FIRE CIDER TONIC

YIELD: ABOUT 40 OUNCES | PREP TIME: 10 MINUTES | INFUSION TIME: 4 TO 6 WEEKS

RECOMMENDED STORAGE: Store in large, sealed glass jars in the refrigerator for up to 1 year.

Fire cider is an old folk remedy that has been used to fight illness and boost the immune system. It is packed with health benefits and a punch of flavor. Its powerhouse ingredients have antibacterial properties, assist with digestion, alleviate sinus congestion, relieve headaches, improve blood circulation, and reduce inflammation and nausea. It is an extremely versatile remedy that can be used for many ailments. Despite the number of ingredients needed, this recipe is quite simple.

½ cup fresh ginger root, peeled and sliced thin

½ cup fresh horseradish, sliced thin

10 garlic cloves, peeled and chopped

1 tablespoon turmeric

1 tablespoon ground cinnamon

2 jalapeño peppers, chopped

2 teaspoons ground black pepper

1 orange, unpeeled and cut into ½-inch pieces

1 lemon, unpeeled and cut into ½-inch pieces

1 small onion, cut into ½-inch pieces

2 to 3 cups apple cider vinegar

¼ cup raw honey

1. Put the ginger, horseradish, garlic, turmeric, cinnamon, jalapeño peppers, and black pepper into a jar, and mash the mixture with a large wooden spoon.

2. Add the orange, lemon, and onion, and mash the mixture again with a large wooden spoon.

3. Pour the apple cider vinegar over the mixture, making sure all the ingredients are submerged.

4. If you are using a jar with a metal lid, put a piece of parchment paper under the lid to avoid a reaction with the vinegar.

5. Store in a cool, dark place for 4 to 6 weeks, shaking the jar for a few seconds every day.

6. After 4 to 6 weeks, strain out the solids and transfer the liquid to a clean jar.

7. Add the raw honey to the liquid and stir until well combined.

USAGE TIP: Fire Cider Tonic has tons of uses. You can take a 2-ounce shot when you feel a cold coming on or to speed the process of beating a cold. You can dilute 2 ounces of the tonic with 8 ounces of water and sip it for a cold-busting beverage. You can also drizzle it on salads or vegetables to enhance the flavor and add nutrients.

EUCALYPTUS SINUS CLEANSER

YIELD: 1 (26-OUNCE) APPLICATION | PREP TIME: 15 MINUTES

RECOMMENDED STORAGE: Storage is not recommended.

I have been making this sinus cleanser for as long as I can remember. When your sinuses are clogged and you are having trouble breathing, this cleanser provides relief and loosens mucus congestion. Eucalyptus is known for its medicinal properties and is associated with clearing chest congestion, suppressing a cough, and breathing easier. This remedy is a game changer!

3 cups water

¼ cup apple cider vinegar

2 to 3 drops eucalyptus essential oil

1. Pour the water into a saucepan and bring to a boil.
2. Remove the boiling water from the heat and carefully pour into a large bowl.
3. Add the apple cider vinegar and eucalyptus oil and gently stir.
4. Put the bowl on a counter and bend over the top of the bowl with a towel over your head and bowl to keep the steam in. Be sure to stand far enough away from the bowl to not burn yourself on the steam but close enough to inhale it. With your eyes closed, breathe in deeply through your nose, inhaling the steam, and slowly exhale through your mouth. Repeat until all the steam is gone.

BONE BROTH LATTE

YIELD: 1 (8-OUNCE) SERVING | PREP TIME: 5 MINUTES | COOK TIME: 10 MINUTES

RECOMMENDED STORAGE: Storage is not recommended.

Bone broth supports digestive health, boosts immune function, strengthens bones, reduces inflammation, and can relieve joint pain. It is can easily be incorporated into your routine and serves so many benefits for your body. This is one of my favorite recipes to make in the morning or afternoon when I want something easy on my stomach but nutrient dense and full of healing benefits. In addition to bone broth, this latte has healthy fats and greens to help support your body's detoxification process.

¾ cup bone broth

¼ cup water

1 cup spinach

2 tablespoons apple cider vinegar

1 tablespoon freshly squeezed lemon juice

1 teaspoon ghee

1 teaspoon coconut oil

1 teaspoon turmeric

Pinch sea salt

Pinch black pepper

1. In a saucepan, combine the bone broth and water. Bring to a simmer over medium-low heat, then remove from heat.

2. Combine the heated bone broth and water mixture, spinach, apple cider vinegar, lemon juice, ghee, coconut oil, turmeric, sea salt, and black pepper in a blender. Blend until smooth.

3. Pour into a mug, sip, and enjoy.

IMMUNITY-BOOSTING GOLDEN LATTE

YIELD: 1 (8-OUNCE) SERVING | PREP TIME: 2 MINUTES | COOK TIME: 10 MINUTES

RECOMMENDED STORAGE: Storage is not recommended.

When your body needs an immunity pick-me-up, this is the perfect cure. It gives you a warm, cozy feeling while delivering plenty of immunity and anti-inflammatory benefits. Turmeric has been used for thousands of years for healing purposes. It contains curcumin, an active ingredient that provides anti-inflammatory effects. Curcumin is also responsible for turmeric's high levels of antioxidants, which protect your body from the free radicals that damage cells and lead to a range of diseases, including cancer. I love this latte as a replacement for coffee in the morning or as a way to wind down in the evening.

½ cup water

½ cup coconut milk

2 tablespoons apple cider vinegar

½ tablespoon turmeric

1 teaspoon honey

Pinch black pepper

1. Put the water, coconut milk, apple cider vinegar, turmeric, honey, and black pepper in a saucepan. Bring to a simmer over medium-low heat.

2. Remove from heat and pour into a mug. Sip and enjoy.

VARIATION TIP: For a frothy latte, as soon as you remove the mixture from the heat, use an immersion blender or a frother in the latte.

DEEP SLEEP SPRAY

YIELD: 8 OUNCES | PREP TIME: 2 MINUTES

RECOMMENDED STORAGE: Store in a glass spray bottle.

Our sense of smell directly correlates with memory and emotion. This makes scents very important when we want to relax, de-stress, and fall asleep easily. Studies have shown that essential oil blends are effective for improving the quality of sleep, even more than individual oils. Sandalwood works to ease anxiety and is known to have sedative effects. Vanilla also has sedative effects, as well as the ability to help reduce restlessness and lower blood pressure. Lavender has been shown to reduce anxiety and aid in pain relief.

¾ cup distilled water

2 tablespoons apple cider vinegar

5 to 7 drops sandalwood essential oil

5 to 7 drops vanilla essential oil

5 to 7 drops lavender essential oil

1. In a reusable spray bottle combine the water, apple cider vinegar, sandalwood essential oil, vanilla essential oil, and lavender essential oil.

2. Cover and shake well.

3. Spray in the air and on wrists as needed.

VARIATION TIP: Sandalwood has also been known to increase alertness. If you find that you are not relaxed while using this spray and instead feel energized, substitute the sandalwood with chamomile.

BLUEBERRY-LAVENDER STRESS-REDUCING SMOOTHIE

YIELD: 1 (16-OUNCE) SERVING | PREP TIME: 5 TO 10 MINUTES

RECOMMENDED STORAGE: Storage is not recommended.

Studies have shown that lavender reduces stress and anxiety while also containing mood-uplifting properties. With the sweet smell and added benefits of vanilla, this smoothie serves as a natural antidepressant, helping to put you in a much better mood. When you are feeling a little down or stressed or just need a mood boost, whip up this deliciously relaxing smoothie.

1 cup almond milk

1 cup spinach

½ frozen banana

½ cup frozen blueberries

2 tablespoons apple cider vinegar

1 teaspoon dried culinary lavender

1 tablespoon chia seeds

1 teaspoon vanilla extract

1. Combine the almond milk, spinach, banana, blueberries, apple cider vinegar, lavender, chia seeds, and vanilla in a blender. Blend until smooth.

2. Pour into a glass, sip, and enjoy.

UNWIND AND RELAX REISHI ELIXIR

YIELD: 1 (8-OUNCE) SERVING | PREP TIME: 5 MINUTES

RECOMMENDED STORAGE: Storage is not recommended.

Reishi mushroom is a medicinal mushroom known for fighting depression, anxiety, and stress. It is an adaptogen, which means it helps the body adapt to stress and has a normalizing effect on the body. It is also high in antioxidants and supports a healthy immune system. This elixir is the perfect way to unwind after a long day. It can even be beneficial midday if you feel like you are experiencing more stress than normal.

1 tablespoon apple cider vinegar

2 teaspoons reishi mushroom powder

1 teaspoon coconut oil

1 cup water

1 teaspoon honey

1. Put the apple cider vinegar, reishi mushroom powder, and coconut oil in a mug.

2. Bring the water to a boil and pour it into the mug, stirring to combine.

3. Stir in the honey with a spoon until fully dissolved. Sip and enjoy.

VARIATION TIP: Add one serving of CBD oil to this elixir. Follow the manufacturer's instructions for the appropriate dose.

MOOD-BOOSTING MOCKTAIL

YIELD: 1 (9-OUNCE) SERVING | PREP TIME: 5 MINUTES

RECOMMENDED STORAGE: Storage is not recommended.

Apple cider vinegar is a natural mood enhancer. When taken before meals, it helps break down proteins into amino acids. This process plays a role in the creation of tryptophan, which is involved in the release of serotonin, the neurotransmitter that makes us feel happy. The addition of probiotics keeps our gut healthy, which is important because about 90 percent of serotonin is made in our digestive tract. This mocktail can be consumed daily to support a happy mood.

1 cup coconut water

3 tablespoons pineapple juice

2 tablespoons apple cider vinegar

1 tablespoon freshly squeezed lemon juice

1 teaspoon honey

1 probiotic capsule

¼ cup sparkling water

1. In a large glass, combine the coconut water, pineapple juice, apple cider vinegar, lemon juice, and honey. Stir with a spoon until well combined.

2. Open the probiotic capsule and empty the contents into the glass.

3. Top off the mixture with sparkling water. (You may not need the full amount.) Lightly stir with a spoon to mix. Sip and enjoy.

ENERGIZING CORDYCEPS LATTE

YIELD: 1 (8-OUNCE) SERVING | PREP TIME: 1 MINUTE | COOK TIME: 5 MINUTES

RECOMMENDED STORAGE: Storage is not recommended.

Cordyceps is a form of medicinal mushrooms that boosts energy and exercise performance. They increase the body's production of ATP (adenosine triphosphate), which delivers energy to the muscles. When combined with apple cider vinegar, they give you just the boost your body needs—without caffeine. This is the perfect caffeine-free way to start your day. It is also a fantastic midday pick-me-up.

1 cup almond milk

1 tablespoon apple cider vinegar

1 teaspoon cordyceps powder

¼ teaspoon apple pie spice

½ teaspoon honey

1. Put the almond milk, apple cider vinegar, cordyceps powder, apple pie spice, and honey in a saucepan set over medium-low heat.

2. Stir frequently until well combined and lightly simmering.

3. Remove from heat, pour into a mug, sip, and enjoy.

HEALTH TIP: Contrary to popular belief, when you are fighting fatigue, you should avoid caffeine and high-glycemic foods. Both cause a spike in blood sugar levels, leading to a boost in energy followed by a crash, rather than sustainable energy.

AFTERNOON PICK-ME-UP TONIC

YIELD: 1 (8-OUNCE) SERVING | PREP TIME: 2 MINUTES

RECOMMENDED STORAGE: Storage is not recommended.

Apple cider vinegar is known as a great replacement for coffee when you are looking for a healthy, noncaffeinated beverage. It is known not only to boost productive energy but also to positively affect immunity and digestion. Combining the vinegar with cinnamon helps balance blood-sugar levels and prevent sugar spikes that lead to a fatigue crash. Cayenne pepper works to boost your metabolism and energy.

1 cup water

1 tablespoon apple cider vinegar

1 tablespoon freshly squeezed lemon juice

¼ teaspoon cinnamon

Dash cayenne pepper

1. Put the water, apple cider vinegar, lemon juice, cinnamon, and cayenne pepper in a glass.

2. Stir the mixture with a spoon until the cinnamon and cayenne pepper are fully incorporated.

3. Consume with a straw and enjoy.

VARIATION TIP: Substitute still water with sparkling water for a fizzy beverage.

LIVER DETOX ELIXIR

YIELD: 1 (8-OUNCE) SERVING | PREP TIME: 5 MINUTES | INFUSION TIME: 10 MINUTES

RECOMMENDED STORAGE: Storage is not recommended.

Studies have shown that milk thistle supports liver health because it contains silymarin, which helps keep toxins from attaching to the liver. It also aids in reducing inflammation and promoting cell repair. Dandelion root supports the liver detoxification process so that your body can correctly filter out toxins and produce hormones. Before or after a night of drinking alcohol, this is a great elixir to support your liver. It can also be consumed regularly to aid in daily liver detoxification.

1 milk thistle tea bag

1 dandelion root tea bag

1 cup water

2 tablespoons apple cider vinegar

¼ teaspoon cinnamon

1 dash nutmeg

1 dash ground ginger

1. Put the milk thistle tea bag and dandelion tea bag in a mug.

2. Bring the water to a boil and pour into the mug. Let steep for 10 minutes.

3. Remove the tea bags and add the apple cider vinegar, cinnamon, nutmeg, and ginger. Stir with a spoon until fully combined. Sip and enjoy.

SIMPLE INSECT REPELLENT

YIELD: 8 OUNCES | PREP TIME: 2 MINUTES

RECOMMENDED STORAGE: Store in a glass spray bottle.

Many insect sprays contain harmful chemicals such as DEET. Studies have shown that DEET can cause neurons in the brain to die, specifically in the learning and memory regions. This can put children at a higher risk of having adverse reactions. Citronella, lemon, and rosemary essential oils all have insect- and mosquito-repellent properties. Apple cider vinegar serves as a great base and is also an insect repellent. The combination of the essential oils and vinegar will be your perfect protection from bites.

¼ cup apple cider vinegar

¼ cup witch hazel

30 drops citronella essential oil

30 drops lemon essential oil

10 drops rosemary essential oil

½ cup water

1. In a glass spray bottle, combine the apple cider vinegar, witch hazel, citronella essential oil, lemon essential oil, and rosemary essential oil. Cover and shake well to combine.

2. Open the spray bottle and add the water. Cover and shake well to combine.

3. Shake well before each use. Spray all over the body (avoiding the eyes) and rub into the skin. Reapply every few hours.

LAVENDER AFTERBITE TREATMENT

YIELD: 4 OUNCES | PREP TIME: 2 MINUTES

RECOMMENDED STORAGE: Store in a glass spray bottle.

This afterbite treatment will help provide natural relief and banish insect bites. The vitamins in aloe vera will reduce the swelling, irritation, and itching associated with insect bites. Apple cider vinegar will help restore the natural pH level of the affected area, providing calmness. Peppermint will provide a cooling effect on the irritated area, creating a soothing feeling. Tea tree essential oil contains antiseptic properties to prevent bacterial infections from a bite.

¼ cup water

¼ cup aloe vera juice

¾ teaspoon apple cider vinegar

3 to 5 drops peppermint essential oil

3 to 5 drops tea tree essential oil

1. In a glass spray bottle, combine the water, aloe vera juice, apple cider vinegar, peppermint essential oil, and tea tree essential oil. Cover and shake well to combine.

2. Shake well before each use. Spray a thin layer onto the bite area and let dry. Apply throughout the day as needed.

BEE STING TREATMENT

YIELD: ABOUT 1 OUNCE, OR 5 APPLICATIONS | PREP TIME: 2 MINUTES

RECOMMENDED STORAGE: Storage is not recommended.

Bee stings are pesky. They result in a sharp pain that leads to discomfort, redness, and swelling. It is best to react as quickly as possible after a bee sting to ensure the fastest relief and recovery. Check to make sure there is no stinger left in your skin. If there is, scrape it out using your fingernail or a credit card. Then sanitize your skin by cleaning it well with soap and water before applying this treatment.

1 tablespoon baking soda

½ tablespoon apple cider vinegar

½ teaspoon raw honey

1 drop tea tree essential oil

1. In a small bowl, stir together the baking soda, apple cider vinegar, raw honey, and tea tree essential oil to make a paste.
2. If the mixture is too thick, add another splash of apple cider vinegar to thin it out so that it is spreadable.
3. Apply a teaspoon of the paste to the area of irritation and let sit for at least 15 minutes.
4. Rinse the paste off with water and reapply as needed.

Aches and Pains

Aches and pains can limit your activities and make every day routines more difficult. This section provides relief for common ailments such as joint pain, cuts, scrapes, bruises, inflammation, and muscle cramps.

FEATURED RECIPES: Aches and Pains Relief Cream (34), Frankincense Joint Relief Massage Oil (35), Carrot-Orange-Ginger Joint Elixir (36), Inflammation-Reducing Golden Smoothie (37), Spicy Ginger Healing Tonic (38), Muscle Cramping Bath Soak (39), Muscle Cramping Oil (40), Eucalyptus-Peppermint Compress (41), Lavender Wound-Healing Salve (42), Chamomile-Rosemary Scrape-Soothing Spray (43), and Bruise Be Gone Solution (44).

ACHES AND PAINS
RELIEF CREAM

**YIELD: 18 OUNCES, OR 108 (TEASPOON-SIZE) APPLICATIONS | PREP TIME: 2 MINUTES
COOK TIME: 5 MINUTES | SET TIME: 5 TO 10 MINUTES**

RECOMMENDED STORAGE: Store in a glass jar at room temperature for up to 1 year.

This cream both warms and cools your body. Cayenne pepper increases circulation and reduces pain by blocking substance P, a neurotransmitter that relays pain to your brain. Peppermint and eucalyptus are anti-inflammatories that calm aches and pains and provide a cooling effect to help relax the muscles.

½ cup hemp seed oil

3 tablespoons apple cider vinegar

3 teaspoons beeswax pastilles

1 tablespoon cayenne pepper

2 teaspoons peppermint essential oil

5 to 7 drops eucalyptus essential oil

1. Put the hemp seed oil, apple cider vinegar, and beeswax in a double boiler on low heat (or a large glass or metal bowl set over a pot of simmering water), stirring with a spoon until the wax is melted.

2. Remove from heat and add the cayenne pepper, peppermint essential oil, and eucalyptus essential oil, stirring with a spoon until well combined.

3. Pour the mixture into a glass jar and allow it to set for about 5 to 10 minutes.

4. To apply, scoop out about 1 teaspoon and rub directly onto the skin. For best results, incorporate with a light massage to relax the muscles.

FRANKINCENSE JOINT RELIEF MASSAGE OIL

YIELD: 8 OUNCES | PREP TIME: 2 MINUTES

RECOMMENDED STORAGE: Store in a glass spray bottle.

This massage oil contains both frankincense and orange essential oils, which play a vital role in easing joint pain and arthritis discomfort. Frankincense works to inhibit the inflammation that is associated with arthritis. It helps prevent the breakdown of cartilage tissue and reduce inflammation. Studies have shown that orange essential oil has positive effects when fighting pain and is known as a natural treatment for arthritis pain.

2 tablespoons apple
cider vinegar

2 tablespoons hemp seed oil

10 drops frankincense
essential oil

10 drops orange essential oil

¼ cup water

1. In a glass spray bottle, combine the apple cider vinegar, hemp seed oil, frankincense essential oil, and orange essential oil.

2. Top off the bottle with the water. (You may not need the full amount.) Cover and shake well to combine.

3. Shake well before each use. Spray a thin layer onto the joint areas that are bothering you and massage for 5 minutes.

CARROT-ORANGE-GINGER JOINT ELIXIR

YIELD: 3 (8-OUNCE) SERVINGS | PREP TIME: 5 MINUTES

RECOMMENDED STORAGE: Store in a large, sealed glass jar in the refrigerator for up to 1 week.

Carrot, orange, and lemon juices are all high in vitamin C and antioxidants, making this a powerhouse combination to fight the inflammation associated with arthritis. Ginger has additional anti-inflammatory properties that help relieve arthritis pain, as well as improve joint function. Magnesium maintains nerve and muscle functions while also strengthening bones. In addition, it works to maintain joint cartilage.

2 carrots

1 orange, peeled

1 lemon, peeled

1 inch fresh ginger root, peeled

2 cups water

2 tablespoons apple cider vinegar

1 tablespoon magnesium citrate powder

1. In a juicer or blender, process the carrots, orange, lemon, and ginger. Discard the pulp if using a juicer.

2. Pour the mixture into a glass jar and add the water, apple cider vinegar, and magnesium citrate powder. Cover and shake well to combine.

3. Consume an 8-ounce cup in the morning.

INFLAMMATION-REDUCING GOLDEN SMOOTHIE

YIELD: 1 (16-OUNCE) SERVING | PREP TIME: 5 MINUTES

RECOMMENDED STORAGE: Store in a large glass in the refrigerator for up to 12 hours.
Longer storage is not recommended.

Pineapple contains bromelain, which is well known for its anti-inflammatory benefits, specifically aiding in the reduction of swelling and bruising. Mango provides additional immune and antioxidant support. Turmeric contains many medicinal properties, including reducing inflammation, boosting brain function, and lowering the risk of certain diseases, such as heart disease. This smoothie is the perfect recipe for reducing inflammation and supporting your body's immune system.

1 cup water

¼ cup frozen pineapple

¼ cup frozen mango

2 tablespoons apple cider vinegar

1 inch fresh ginger root, peeled

¼ teaspoon ground turmeric

½ frozen banana (optional)

1. Combine the water, pineapple, mango, apple cider vinegar, ginger, turmeric, and banana (if using) in a blender. Blend until smooth.

2. If the mixture is too thick, add a splash of water at a time, and blend until it reaches your desired consistency.

3. Pour into a cup and enjoy.

SPICY GINGER HEALING TONIC

**YIELD: 1 (8-OUNCE) SERVING | PREP TIME: 1 MINUTE | COOK TIME: 5 MINUTES
INFUSION TIME: 10 MINUTES**

RECOMMENDED STORAGE: Storage is not recommended.

Ginger has been widely used in Ayurvedic medicine to treat headaches and migraines. Cayenne pepper contains capsaicin, which helps block the neurotransmitters responsible for sending pain signals to the brain. This tonic can be used for headache prevention or to help ease the pain from headaches and migraines.

1 cup water

1 ginger tea bag

2 tablespoons apple cider vinegar

¼ teaspoon cayenne pepper

1 teaspoon raw honey (optional)

1. Pour the water into a saucepan and heat on the stove until boiling.
2. Remove from heat and add the ginger tea bag.
3. Cover the saucepan and infuse for 10 minutes.
4. Remove the tea bag and add the apple cider vinegar, cayenne pepper, and honey (if using).
5. Stir until combined. Sip and enjoy.

MUSCLE CRAMPING BATH SOAK

YIELD: 1 TREATMENT | PREP TIME: 10 MINUTES

Muscle cramping is common mid- or post-exercise. It is often caused by tight muscles, dehydration, or electrolyte depletion. Soaking in a hot bath with apple cider vinegar, chamomile, and eucalyptus will help increase blood flow and allow the muscles to relax. It is very important to properly hydrate both before and after the bath to prevent future cramping.

½ cup Epsom salt

⅓ cup apple cider vinegar

10 drops chamomile essential oil

5 to 7 drops eucalyptus essential oil

1. Draw a warm bath.
2. Add the Epsom salt, apple cider vinegar, chamomile essential oil, and eucalyptus essential oil to the bath water.
3. Give everything a big swirl in the tub to mix.
4. Soak in the bath for at least 20 minutes for best results.

USAGE TIP: Light stretching in the tub will enhance results. Hold stretches for 20 to 30 seconds at a time. The combination of heat and stretching will help decrease muscle spasms and increase blood flow.

MUSCLE CRAMPING OIL

YIELD: 8 OUNCES | PREP TIME: 2 MINUTES

RECOMMENDED STORAGE: Store in a glass spray bottle.

This oil is perfect for massaging into the skin when you experience muscle cramping after a workout. You can also apply it before a workout to prevent cramping. Clary sage has been shown to alleviate both muscle spasms and tension. Arnica and lemongrass essential oils relieve inflammation, which is often a precursor to muscle cramping. They also reduce swelling while soothing the skin.

2 tablespoons apple cider vinegar

2 tablespoons hemp seed oil

15 drops clary sage essential oil

15 drops arnica essential oil

7 drops lemongrass essential oil

¼ cup water

1. In a glass spray bottle, combine the apple cider vinegar, hemp seed oil, clary sage essential oil, arnica essential oil, and lemongrass essential oil.

2. Top off the bottle with the water. (You may not need the full amount.) Cover and shake well to combine.

3. Shake well before each use and spray a thin layer on your feet and the back of your neck.

EUCALYPTUS-PEPPERMINT COMPRESS

YIELD: 8 OUNCES | PREP TIME: 1 MINUTE | COOK TIME: 5 MINUTES | TREATMENT TIME: 20 MINUTES

RECOMMENDED STORAGE: Storage is not recommended.

Apple cider vinegar works to reduce inflammation and swelling in the joints. Eucalyptus helps reduce pain, swelling, and inflammation, and peppermint adds a cooling effect that relaxes muscles and eases pain and spasms. This compress is perfect for sore muscles, pulled muscles, and general pain.

½ cup water

½ cup apple cider vinegar

5 to 7 drops eucalyptus essential oil

5 to 7 drops peppermint essential oil

2 clean hand towels

1. In a small saucepan, combine the water and apple cider vinegar and heat on low until warm.

2. Add the eucalyptus essential oil and the peppermint essential oil, stirring to combine. Remove from heat.

3. Soak two clean hand towels in the warm mixture and wring out excess liquid.

4. Wrap the hand towels wherever you are sore and achy, and let sit for 20 minutes.

LAVENDER WOUND-HEALING SALVE

YIELD: 18 OUNCES, OR 108 (1-TEASPOON) APPLICATIONS | PREP TIME: 2 MINUTES
COOK TIME: 5 TO 10 MINUTES | SET TIME: 5 TO 10 MINUTES

RECOMMENDED STORAGE: Store in a glass jar at room temperature for up to 1 year.

Lavender essential oil is extremely effective when it comes to healing wounds because it can increase cell growth, leading to a faster healing time. Tea tree essential oil is an antiseptic and anti-inflammatory that helps relieve and soothe painful wounds. While the skin is healing, oregano and rosemary essential oils work to protect it from additional bacterial infections.

1¾ cups hemp seed oil

¼ cup apple cider vinegar

12 drops lavender essential oil

8 drops tea tree essential oil

5 drops oregano essential oil

5 drops rosemary essential oil

¼ cup beeswax pastilles

1. Put the hemp seed oil, apple cider vinegar, lavender essential oil, tea tree essential oil, oregano essential oil, and rosemary essential oil in a bowl, stirring with a spoon to combine.

2. Heat the beeswax in a double boiler over low heat (or a large glass or metal bowl set over a pot of simmering water), stirring with a spoon until melted.

3. Turn off the heat and add the hemp seed oil mixture, stirring with a spoon until well combined.

4. Pour the mixture into a glass jar and let it set for about 5 to 10 minutes.

5. Once it is set, gently dab the salve onto the wound, making sure it covers the entire area. You can apply regularly until the wound is healed.

CHAMOMILE-ROSEMARY SCRAPE-SOOTHING SPRAY

YIELD: 6 OUNCES | PREP TIME: 5 MINUTES

RECOMMENDED STORAGE: Store in a glass spray bottle.

Chamomile is known for its soothing and healing properties. When applied topically, it has anti-inflammatory and antimicrobial properties that work to speed up the healing process and provide relief. Rosemary essential oil, tea tree essential oil, and apple cider vinegar reduce inflammation and kill bacteria to heal scrapes and cuts. Hemp seed oil strengthens the skin to fight off bacterial and viral infections.

¼ apple cider vinegar

10 drops chamomile essential oil

10 drops rosemary essential oil

5 drops tea tree essential oil

½ cup hemp seed oil

1. In a glass spray bottle, combine the apple cider vinegar, chamomile essential oil, rosemary essential oil, and tea tree essential oil. Cover and shake well to combine.

2. Open the bottle and add the hemp seed oil. Cover and shake well to combine.

3. Shake well before each use, and spray several pumps daily onto cuts, scrapes, and rashes.

VARIATION TIP: Substitute jojoba oil or almond oil for the hemp seed oil.

BRUISE BE GONE SOLUTION

YIELD: 45 TO 55 (TEASPOON-SIZE) APPLICATIONS | PREP TIME: 2 MINUTES
COOK TIME: 10 MINUTES

RECOMMENDED STORAGE: Store in a tin or glass jar.

This solution works wonders to reduce the appearance of bruises. Vitamin C and hemp seed oil contain powerful anti-inflammatory properties, and comfrey oil has been used in European and Japanese cultures for thousands of years for its healing properties. It is specifically known for its use in the treatment of bruises, muscle sprains, burns, and inflammation. This cream can be used at the first sight of a bruise and applied regularly until the bruise has disappeared.

½ cup shea butter

¼ cup hemp seed oil

¼ cup apple cider vinegar

4 to 5 drops comfrey oil

4 vitamin C capsules

1. Heat the shea butter and hemp seed oil in a double boiler (or a large glass or metal bowl set over a pot of simmering water) until melted, stirring occasionally.

2. Remove from heat and add the apple cider vinegar and comfrey oil.

3. Open the vitamin C capsules and pour the contents into the shea butter mixture, stirring until fully dissolved.

4. Pour the mixture into a reusable jar and let it set for 10 to 15 minutes.

5. When you are ready to use the solution, scoop out a teaspoon-size amount, warm it in your hands, and gently massage the bruised area.

USAGE TIP: Although the cream will take several hours to fully set, it can also be used as a liquid.

HEALTH TIP: To heal bruises even faster, apply an ice pack immediately after the injury. This will help reduce blood flow and prevent the bruise from swelling and becoming as dark.

Digestion

Issues with our digestive systems can be chronic or occasional. The recipes in this section are designed to relieve indigestion, heartburn, bloating, constipation, and nausea due to motion sickness.

FEATURED RECIPES: Pumpkin Pie Digestive Gummies (46), De-bloat Sipper (47), Morning Digestion Tonic (48), Stay Regular Morning Tonic (49), Regular Digestion Shooter (50), Orange-Ginger Constipation Bites (51), Heartburn Sipper (52), Acid Reflux Tea (53), Happy Gut Smoothie (54), and Motion Sickness Gummies (55).

PUMPKIN PIE DIGESTIVE GUMMIES

YIELD: 12 (1-OUNCE) SERVINGS | PREP TIME: 10 MINUTES
COOK TIME: 5 MINUTES | SET TIME: 2 HOURS

RECOMMENDED STORAGE: Store in the refrigerator for up to one week.

SPECIAL MATERIALS NEEDED: Candy mold, silicone ice cube tray, or glass baking dish.

Increasing our intake of foods that have gut-healing properties is one of the best things we can do for our bodies and digestive systems. These gummies are a super simple and fun way to boost gut healing. Gelatin helps the lining of the gut to heal and the stomach to produce digestive enzymes, which can lessen symptoms such as indigestion, bloating, heartburn, and acid reflux.

⅔ cup water

⅓ cup apple cider vinegar

2 teaspoons pumpkin pie spice

1 teaspoon maple syrup

3 tablespoons gelatin

1 teaspoon coconut oil (if using a glass baking dish)

1. Put the water, apple cider vinegar, and pumpkin pie spice in a saucepan and whisk together until well combined.

2. Warm the liquid over medium heat.

3. Remove from heat when it is warm but not boiling.

4. Add the maple syrup and stir until dissolved.

5. Sprinkle the gelatin evenly over the liquid while stirring to ensure that it dissolves.

6. After all the gelatin is incorporated, pour the mixture into a candy mold or silicone ice cube tray. You can also use a glass baking dish greased with coconut oil.

7. Refrigerate the gummies for at least two hours until set.

DE-BLOAT SIPPER

YIELD: 1 (8-OUNCE) SERVING | PREP TIME: 15 MINUTES

RECOMMENDED STORAGE: Storage is not recommended.

Bloating is an uncomfortable feeling. Your stomach expands, and it usually takes a while to bring it back down to normal. Bloating can be caused by anything from digestive stress, allergic reactions to food, excess gas, parasites, or an imbalance of intestinal bacteria. This sipper works to reduce inflammation, decrease fluid retention, and calm the stomach, while hydrating you so that you can reduce bloating faster and feel energized. Celery helps support the digestive tract and decreases fluid retention in the body, which in turn reduces bloating.

1 large stalk celery, chopped into 1-inch pieces

1 cucumber, sliced

1 inch fresh ginger root, peeled

2 tablespoons apple cider vinegar

Juice of ½ lemon

1. Combine the celery, cucumber, and ginger root in a blender. Blend until smooth.

2. Strain the mixture through cheesecloth or a fine mesh strainer.

3. Pour the strained mixture into a cup and stir in the apple cider vinegar and lemon juice until well combined.

4. Consume immediately.

HEALTH TIP: If you are experiencing bloating, take a probiotic with this beverage to help restore healthy bacteria to your gut and aid in a healthy digestion process.

MORNING DIGESTION TONIC

YIELD: 1 (9-OUNCE) SERVING | PREP TIME: 1 MINUTE | COOK TIME: 5 MINUTES

RECOMMENDED STORAGE: Storage is not recommended.

Morning is the perfect opportunity to set the tone for your digestive system. What you consume in the morning affects the rest of your day. By starting the day with apple cider vinegar and lemon, you are boosting your immune system with vitamin C, getting your digestive system moving, and telling your stomach to start producing enzymes to digest the first meal of the day. The addition of cayenne pepper gives your metabolism a boost first thing in the morning, aiding in weight loss.

1 cup water

2 tablespoons apple cider vinegar

Juice of ½ lemon

Dash cayenne pepper

1. On the stove, heat the water in a saucepan until warm but not hot.

2. Remove from heat and add the apple cider vinegar, lemon juice, and cayenne pepper.

3. Pour into a mug and consume immediately.

STAY REGULAR MORNING TONIC

YIELD: 1 (10-OUNCE) SERVING | PREP: 5 MINUTES | SET TIME: 10 TO 15 MINUTES

RECOMMENDED STORAGE: Store in a glass jar for up to 5 days in the refrigerator.

Chia seeds are the star ingredient in this morning tonic. They contain soluble fiber, which helps relieve constipation. The key is to let them "gel" so that they do not cause any digestive issues. Cucumber and lemon juice both work to hydrate you and support regular bowel movements.

1 cup water

1 cucumber, sliced

Juice of ½ lemon

2 tablespoons apple cider vinegar

2 tablespoons chia seeds

1. Put the water, cucumber, lemon juice, apple cider vinegar, and chia seeds in a blender. Blend until smooth.

2. Pour into a cup and refrigerate for 5 minutes.

3. Stir the tonic and refrigerate for another 5 to 10 minutes for the chia seeds to gel.

4. Stir one final time with a spoon, sip, and enjoy.

PREPARATION TIP: Make this tonic the night before and refrigerate overnight so that it is ready first thing in the morning.

REGULAR DIGESTION SHOOTER

YIELD: 1 (4-OUNCE) SERVING | PREP TIME: 2 MINUTES

PREPARATION TIP: Make in a large quantity for the week so that every morning you can wake up and stimulate your digestive system.

Prune juice is a well-known remedy for constipation. It stimulates bowel movements and may help prevent colon cancer. Prune juice can also help control diabetes and obesity, and is a great source of iron and potassium. When combined with apple cider vinegar and lemon juice, prune juice gives your gastrointestinal tract the push it needs. Make sure to consume a large glass of water after taking this shooter. When it comes to being regular, hydration is of utmost importance.

¼ cup prune juice

2 tablespoons apple cider vinegar

Juice of 1 lemon

1. Put the prune juice, apple cider vinegar, and lemon juice in a small glass and stir until combined.

2. Consume no more than three times per day for up to one week. Take a break for at least one week before resuming.

ORANGE-GINGER CONSTIPATION BITES

YIELD: APPROXIMATELY 25 (2-OUNCE) SERVINGS | PREP TIME: 10 MINUTES | SET TIME: 1 HOUR

RECOMMENDED STORAGE: Store in an airtight container in the refrigerator for up to two weeks.

SPECIAL MATERIALS NEEDED: Silicone candy mold.

Constipation can stem from poor digestion, which is why it is vital to eat foods that support a healthy digestive process when you are suffering from constipation. Psyllium husk is known to help increase bowel movements and relieve chronic constipation. Ginger is a natural laxative, making it an extremely effective treatment for constipation. Ginger also helps strengthen the stomach, promote digestion, and stimulate appetite. These chews are great to have when you are experiencing constipation and bloating.

1 cup organic extra virgin coconut oil, melted

2 tablespoons orange juice

2 tablespoons freshly squeezed lemon juice

2 tablespoons apple cider vinegar

2 tablespoons honey

2 tablespoons psyllium husk

1 teaspoon fresh ginger root, grated

¼ teaspoon sea salt

1. Put the melted coconut oil, orange juice, lemon juice, apple cider vinegar, honey, psyllium husk, ginger, and sea salt in a blender. Blend until smooth.

2. Pour even amounts into a silicone candy mold.

3. Freeze for 1 hour until set.

PREPARATION TIP: Put the candy mold in the freezer ahead of time to make the removal process easier.

HEARTBURN SIPPER

YIELD: 1 (9-OUNCE) SERVING | PREP TIME: 5 MINUTES | INFUSION TIME: 5 MINUTES

RECOMMENDED STORAGE: Store in the refrigerator for up to 5 days. Reheat on low heat on the stove when you are ready to consume.

Chamomile tea is known for easing and calming an irritated digestive system. It can help prevent acid reflux, which leads to heartburn. Ginger works to lower inflammation and decrease acid reflux by reducing the acid flowing from the stomach back into the esophagus. It is also high in antioxidants and promotes healthy digestion.

1 cup water

1 bag chamomile tea

2 tablespoons apple cider vinegar

2 tablespoons fresh ginger root, grated

Juice of ½ lemon

1. Bring the water to a boil and pour over the chamomile tea in a mug. Steep for about 5 minutes.
2. Add the apple cider vinegar, ginger, and lemon juice to the mug and stir to combine.
3. Sip and enjoy.

ACID REFLUX TEA

YIELD: 1 (8-OUNCE) SERVING | PREP TIME: 1 MINUTE
INFUSION TIME: 10 MINUTES

RECOMMENDED STORAGE: Store in the refrigerator for up to 5 days.

Acid reflux is often caused by a lack of acid balance in the stomach, which causes stomach acid to leak back into the esophagus. Licorice root calms the effects of stomach acid by increasing the mucus that coats the esophageal lining. It can also increase the repair rate of the stomach lining. Apple cider vinegar works to restore the balance of acid in the stomach, aiding the digestive process and reducing acid reflux. This tea is great to drink before a meal to prepare your body for digesting food and to prevent acid reflux.

1 cup water

1 teaspoon licorice root tea

2 tablespoons apple cider vinegar

1. Pour the water into a pot and bring to a boil on the stove.
2. Remove from heat and add the licorice root tea. Cover the pot and let sit for 10 minutes.
3. Strain out the licorice root and pour the tea into a mug.
4. Stir in the apple cider vinegar. Sip and enjoy.

HAPPY GUT SMOOTHIE

YIELD: 1 (16-OUNCE) SERVING | PREP TIME: 5 MINUTES

RECOMMENDED STORAGE: Storage is not recommended.

The gut is known as the second brain. It is in charge of producing hormones and regulating many functions of the body. Keeping your gut healthy is one of the most important things you can do to support your mood, immune system, and digestive health. Collagen supports a healthy gut barrier and is extremely beneficial for digestion. Flax seeds increase good bacteria and fatty acids, and studies have shown that they help relieve inflammation in the colon. This smoothie contains a range of gut-supporting ingredients so that you can have a healthy, happy gut.

2 cups spinach

1 cup coconut milk

½ frozen banana

2 tablespoons apple cider vinegar

2 tablespoons collagen powder

1 tablespoon hemp hearts

½ tablespoon sprouted flax seeds

1 teaspoon cinnamon

1 teaspoon vanilla bean powder, or 1 teaspoon vanilla extract

1. Put the spinach, coconut milk, banana, apple cider vinegar, collagen powder, hemp hearts, flax seeds, cinnamon, and vanilla bean powder into a blender. Blend until smooth.

2. If the smoothie is too thick, add one splash of water at a time, and blend until the desired consistency is reached.

3. Pour into a glass, sip, and enjoy.

MOTION SICKNESS GUMMIES

YIELD: 12 (1-OUNCE) SERVINGS | PREP TIME: 10 MINUTES
COOK TIME: 10 MINUTES | SET TIME: 2 HOURS

RECOMMENDED STORAGE: Store in the refrigerator for up to one week.

SPECIAL MATERIALS NEEDED: Candy mold, glass baking dish, or silicone ice cube tray.

With motion sickness comes nausea, vomiting, and dizziness. Studies have shown that licorice root significantly decreases symptoms of nausea and dyspepsia. These gummies will help prevent and reduce the symptoms of motion sickness. They are perfect to bring with you when you know you are going to drive in a car, fly in a plane, ride on a boat, or do anything else that induces your motion sickness.

1 teaspoon coconut oil
(if using a baking dish)

⅔ cup brewed
licorice root tea

⅓ cup apple cider vinegar

2 teaspoons fresh ginger
root, peeled and minced

1 teaspoon honey

3 tablespoons gelatin

1. If you are using a baking dish, grease it with coconut oil and set aside.

2. In a saucepan, whisk together the licorice root tea, apple cider vinegar, ginger root, and honey until well combined.

3. Warm the mixture over medium heat and remove it from heat before it boils.

4. Sprinkle the gelatin evenly over the liquid while stirring to ensure that it dissolves.

5. Once all the gelatin is mixed in, pour the mixture into the baking dish, candy mold, or ice cube tray.

6. Refrigerate the gummies for at least 2 hours until set.

7. Cut into 12 equal portions if using a baking dish.

8. Eat as needed. No more than 6 per day.

Women's Health

At certain times of the month or at different stages in life, women can encounter some difficult and unpleasant symptoms. The recipes in this section tackle menstruation cramps, morning sickness, and hot flashes.

FEATURED RECIPES: PMS Balance Massage Butter (57), PMS Ease Tea (58), Peppermint Stomach Cramp Tonic (59), Ginger Morning Sickness Mocktail (60), Maternity Rescue Spray (61), Hot Flash Relaxing Oil (62), and Cooling Relief Spray (63).

PMS BALANCE MASSAGE BUTTER

YIELD: 40 TO 50 (TEASPOON-SIZE) APPLICATIONS | PREP TIME: 15 MINUTES
COOK TIME: 10 MINUTES

RECOMMENDED STORAGE: Store in a tin or a glass jar.

This massage butter contains both lavender and chamomile, two essential oils that play a vital role in easing menstruation cramps and discomfort. Lavender improves blood flow to reduce cramps and aids in calming the mind. Chamomile, along with apple cider vinegar, has anti-inflammatory properties that help relax muscles and ease pain. This butter can be used as a preventive measure or when discomfort begins. It can be used multiple times a day as needed until cramps and pain subside.

1 cup shea butter

3 tablespoons apple cider vinegar

40 drops lavender essential oil

20 drops chamomile essential oil

1. Heat the shea butter on medium-low in a double boiler (or in a large glass or metal bowl set over a pot of simmering water) until melted.

2. Remove from heat and add the apple cider vinegar, lavender essential oil, and chamomile essential oil.

3. Stir with a spoon until fully mixed.

4. Pour the mixture into a reusable tin or jar.

5. When you are ready to use, scoop out a teaspoon-size amount, warm it in your hands, and gently massage it into the area that is cramping.

USAGE TIP: Although the butter will take several hours to fully set, it can also be used as a liquid.

PMS EASE TEA

YIELD: 1 (8-OUNCE) SERVING | PREP TIME: 5 MINUTES | INFUSION TIME: 5 MINUTES

RECOMMENDED STORAGE: Storage is not recommended.

Chamomile tea is known for reducing menstrual cramps because it inhibits prostaglandins. Prostaglandins are responsible for major uterus cramps, pain, nausea, vomiting, and diarrhea. Chamomile combined with cinnamon can help reduce pain, bleeding, and nausea. Apple cider vinegar will reduce general cramping by relaxing the muscles that tighten during this process.

1 cup water

1 bag chamomile tea

1 tablespoon apple cider vinegar

½ teaspoon cinnamon

½ teaspoon raw honey

1. Boil the water and pour over the tea bag into a mug. Steep for about 5 minutes.

2. Add the apple cider vinegar, cinnamon, and raw honey to the brewed tea.

3. Stir with a spoon, sip, and enjoy.

PEPPERMINT STOMACH CRAMP TONIC

YIELD: 2 (8-OUNCE) SERVINGS | PREP TIME: 2 MINUTES

RECOMMENDED STORAGE: Store in a large jar for no more than 48 hours.

This sipping tonic has the perfect blend of cramp-easing ingredients. Lemon is a diuretic, which increases the passing of urine, in turn reducing bloating. Mint is an anti-inflammatory that helps calm the stomach and ease digestion.

2 teaspoons apple cider vinegar

Juice of ½ lemon

5 to 6 mint leaves

2 cups water

1. In a jar, combine the apple cider vinegar, lemon juice, and mint leaves.

2. Add the water and stir with a spoon.

3. Seal the jar and put it in the refrigerator for at least 2 hours.

HEALTH TIP: When experiencing cramps, consuming plenty of water is key.

GINGER MORNING SICKNESS MOCKTAIL

YIELD: 1 (16-OUNCE) SERVING | PREP TIME: 5 MINUTES | COOK TIME: 15 MINUTES

RECOMMENDED STORAGE: Store in the refrigerator for up to 5 days.

Ginger has been used in healing for over two thousand years. It has natural nausea-reducing effects that are very beneficial for pregnant women experiencing morning sickness. Consuming this tea once or twice per day can help ease morning sickness and general nausea. Combined with apple cider vinegar, ginger helps reduce any inflammation-causing discomfort. Fresh lemon juice provides a boost of vitamin C to keep your immune system functioning properly.

1½ cups water

1 inch fresh ginger root, peeled and thinly sliced

2 tablespoons apple cider vinegar

½ tablespoon freshly squeezed lemon juice

1. Put the water in a small pot. Add the ginger and bring to a boil.
2. Reduce the heat to medium-low and simmer for 10 minutes.
3. Remove from heat and add the apple cider vinegar and lemon juice.
4. Pour into a mug, sip, and enjoy.

MATERNITY RESCUE SPRAY

YIELD: 8 OUNCES | PREP TIME: 2 MINUTES

RECOMMENDED STORAGE: Store in a glass spray bottle.

This essential oil spray is the perfect pick-me-up for days with morning sickness and pregnancy-induced nausea. Studies have shown that the combination of ginger and citrus can significantly reduce pregnancy-induced nausea and sickness. Spray around your body in the morning, afternoon, or evening for a soothing, uplifting boost that calms an upset stomach.

¾ cup distilled water

3 tablespoons apple cider vinegar

2 tablespoons jojoba oil

3 to 4 drops ginger essential oil

3 to 4 drops orange essential oil

2 to 3 drops lemon essential oil

1. Put the water, apple cider vinegar, jojoba oil, ginger essential oil, orange essential oil, and lemon essential oil in a reusable spray bottle. Cover and shake well to combine.

2. Spray in the air and on wrists as needed.

USAGE TIP: This mixture is also great to spray on bed linens or in the car for a refreshing welcome.

HOT FLASH RELAXING OIL

YIELD: 8 OUNCES | PREP TIME: 2 MINUTES

RECOMMENDED STORAGE: Store in a glass spray bottle.

This oil helps balance hormone levels, boost your mood, and reduce stress and the discomfort of hot flashes. Sandalwood essential oil has a grounding and cooling effect that works to calm hot flashes. Basil essential oil is known as a hormone-balancing oil that can help the body adapt to changing hormones. Lavender induces feelings of relaxation and improves mood. It can help improve sleep quality and ease feelings of discomfort.

2 tablespoons apple cider vinegar

2 tablespoons hemp seed oil

15 drops sandalwood essential oil

15 drops basil essential oil

7 drops lavender essential oil

¼ cup water

1. In a glass spray bottle, combine the apple cider vinegar, hemp seed oil, sandalwood essential oil, basil essential oil, and lavender essential oil.

2. Top off the bottle with the water. (You may not need the full amount.) Cover and shake well to combine.

3. Shake well before each use and spray a thin layer on your feet and the back of your neck.

COOLING RELIEF SPRAY

YIELD: 6 OUNCES | PREP TIME: 2 MINUTES

RECOMMENDED STORAGE: Store in a glass spray bottle.

This cooling spray provides the perfect relief for hot flashes. Apple cider vinegar and witch hazel contain astringent and cooling properties. Geranium essential oil helps calm stress levels and alleviate mood swings. Clary sage essential oil has been known to help with hormonal issues and reduce the frequency of hot flashes. Peppermint essential oil provides a cooling effect that also gives your mood a boost.

¼ cup apple cider vinegar

15 drops geranium essential oil

15 drops clary sage essential oil

7 drops peppermint essential oil

½ cup witch hazel

1. In a glass spray bottle, combine the apple cider vinegar, geranium essential oil, clary sage essential oil, and peppermint essential oil. Cover and shake well to combine.

2. Open the bottle and top off with the witch hazel. (You may not need the full amount.) Cover and shake well to combine.

3. Shake well before each use, and spray on your body to reduce the intensity of hot flashes.

USAGE TIP: This spray is also great to use after a workout or a hot day in the sun to help your body cool down and feel refreshed.

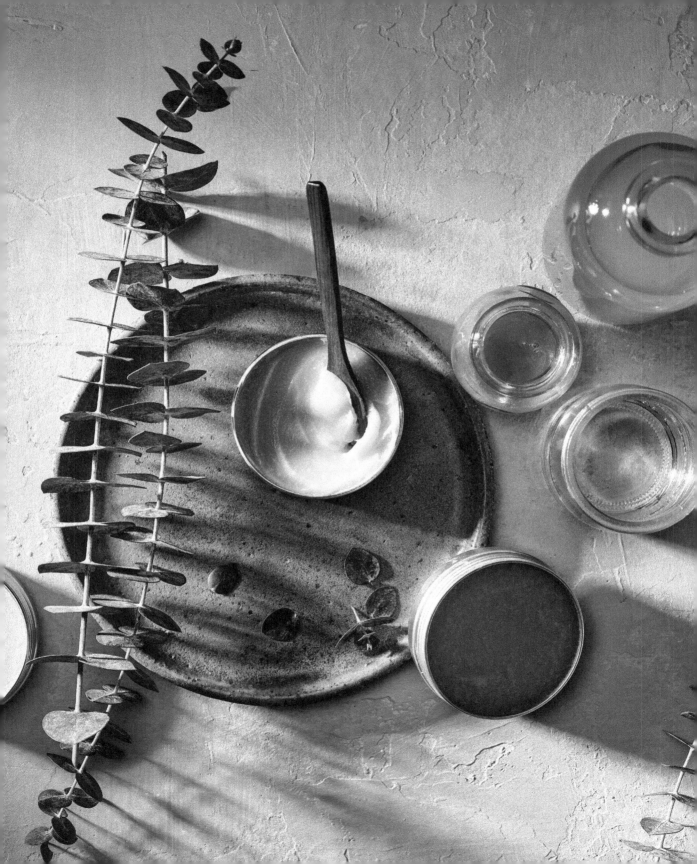

CHAPTER 3

Beauty

You may have noticed, apple cider vinegar has taken over the beauty world. It contains beneficial acids, vitamins, and minerals that make it a beauty powerhouse. In this chapter, a wealth of recipes delve into apple cider vinegar's uses for skin, hair, and nails. Rather than spending a fortune on department store and designer beauty products, try these easy recipes with items from your pantry.

Skin

As our largest organ, skin comes with a seemingly endless number of possible problems and time-consuming maintenance. This section provides simple and natural recipes to address acne, dry skin, eczema, foot care, hand and nail care, hyperpigmentation, ingrown hairs, lips, underarms, varicose veins, and sunburn.

FEATURED RECIPES: Calming Chamomile Acne Body Spray (67), Basic Acne-Clearing Skin Toner (68), Tea Tree Acne Spot Treatment (69), Acne-Healing Clay Mask (70), Avocado Honey Mask (71), Cucumber Makeup-Setting Spray (72), Rose Water Hydrating Skin Spritz (73), Healing Carrot Seed Serum (74), Oatmeal-Honey Bath Soak (75), Magnesium-Salt Spray (76), Simple Green Alkaline Smoothie (77), Tea Tree and Clove Antifungal Foot Soak (78), Athlete's Foot Probiotic Salve (79), Soothing Peppermint Foot Scrub (80), Eucalyptus Hand-Repair Cream (81), Brittle Nail Recovery Treatment (82), Pumpkin Pie Hand Scrub (83), Lemon-Sandalwood Toner (84), Pineapple Enzyme Mask (85), Apple Pie Brightening Skin Mask (86), Lavender-Lemon Ingrown-Hair Spray (87), Ingrown Hair–Fighting Sugar Scrub (88), Peppermint-Vanilla Lip Scrub (89), Grapefruit-Thyme Underarm Detox Treatment (90), Geranium-Cypress Varicose Vein Spray (91), Lemon-Ginger Varicose Vein Massage Oil (92), Chamomile-Sage Varicose Vein Bath Soak (93), Lavender-Oatmeal Sunburn Soak (94), Sunburn Healing Spray (95), and Hydrating Sunburn Tonic (96).

CALMING CHAMOMILE ACNE BODY SPRAY

YIELD: 8 OUNCES | PREP TIME: 2 MINUTES

RECOMMENDED STORAGE: Store in a glass spray bottle.

Chamomile is loaded with antioxidants and calming agents. It nourishes the skin, fights acne, and accelerates the healing process without drying or irritating the skin. Apple cider vinegar works to kill bacteria on the skin, remove dead skin cells, and help prevent future breakouts. Geranium essential oil has been used for thousands of years for its healing properties. It helps balance the production of oil in the skin, reduce inflammation, and increase wound healing. In combination, these ingredients become an acne-fighting machine. Use this body spray daily to both prevent acne and help it heal faster when breakouts on the skin do happen.

1 cup brewed and cooled chamomile tea

2 tablespoons apple cider vinegar

2 tablespoons witch hazel

3 to 4 drops geranium essential oil

1. In a reusable spray bottle, combine the chamomile tea, apple cider vinegar, witch hazel, and geranium essential oil.

2. Shake well before each use, and spray on skin as needed.

USAGE TIP: This spray is perfect to use before exercising to prevent back breakouts, and also after exercising if you cannot shower right away.

BASIC ACNE-CLEARING SKIN TONER

YIELD: 8 OUNCES | PREP TIME: 2 MINUTES

RECOMMENDED STORAGE: Store in a glass container in the refrigerator.

Our skin is naturally acidic. When we use harsh cleansers and soaps, our natural acidity is disrupted. Apple cider vinegar is ideal for skin because it restores that natural acidity and balances the skin's pH level, making the skin both less oily and less dry. It also helps remove excess makeup and dirt and kills acne-causing bacteria. When used daily, this toner can help prevent breakouts, as well as heal current breakouts faster. It also helps reduce the redness and irritation associated with acne.

1 cup distilled water

2 tablespoons apple cider vinegar

1. Combine the water and apple cider vinegar in a reusable glass bottle. Cover and shake well.
2. Pour a small amount onto a cotton pad, and gently apply to your skin after cleansing. Be sure to avoid your eyes.

HEALTH TIP: Moisturizing is crucial when experiencing breakouts. Make sure to follow your toning routine with a non-pore-clogging moisturizer.

TEA TREE ACNE SPOT TREATMENT

YIELD: 2 OUNCES | PREP TIME: 2 MINUTES

RECOMMENDED STORAGE: Store in a sealed glass jar in the refrigerator.

Aloe vera gel is well-known for its healing benefits and its ability to calm the skin. It also contains vitamins A, C, E, and B_{12}, which provide antiaging properties. Tea tree essential oil possesses many antibacterial and antimicrobial properties. It fights inflammation, calms redness, and helps reduce acne scars. If you have a breakout, immediately apply this spot treatment. The faster you take action, the faster your breakout can heal.

¼ cup aloe vera gel

2 tablespoons apple cider vinegar

10 drops tea tree essential oil

1. Put the aloe vera gel, apple cider vinegar, and tea tree essential oil in a glass jar and stir until well combined.

2. To apply, dip a clean cotton swab in the spot treatment and gently dab on affected areas after cleansing. Let it sit overnight and wash off in the morning.

HEALTH TIP: Test this spot treatment on a small patch of your skin before applying to your face to make sure you do not have a reaction to tea tree essential oil.

INGREDIENT TIP: Make sure to purchase 100 percent therapeutic grade tea tree essential oil that is certified organic. You want to put the best possible product on your skin, not one that includes fillers or additives.

ACNE-HEALING CLAY MASK

YIELD: 1 APPLICATION | PREP TIME: 2 MINUTES

RECOMMENDED STORAGE: Storage is not recommended.

Bentonite clay is made from minerals such as iron, sodium, calcium, potassium, and magnesium. It detoxifies and clarifies the skin, helping to both unclog and shrink pores. It also helps control the overproduction of sebum and removes dead skin cells that are big acne causers. Raw honey is loaded with antioxidants and antibacterial properties. It naturally opens the pores so the rest of the ingredients can do their work. This mask has been a staple in my routine for years. I use it not only to prevent breakouts but also to help breakouts heal faster when they do occur.

2 tablespoons apple cider vinegar

1 to 2 tablespoons water

1 tablespoon bentonite clay

1 tablespoon raw honey (preferably manuka)

1. Put the apple cider vinegar, water, bentonite clay, and raw honey in a small bowl.

2. Mix all the ingredients until thoroughly combined. The mixture will fizz a bit at first.

3. After cleansing your face, apply to the skin (avoiding your eyes) and leave for 10 to 15 minutes.

4. To remove the mask, wash your face with lukewarm water and a washcloth.

HEALTH TIP: Be sure to use your favorite moisturizer containing non-pore-clogging ingredients afterward. It will help seal in the active ingredients from the mask and prevent water loss in the skin.

AVOCADO HONEY MASK

YIELD: 1 APPLICATION | PREP TIME: 5 MINUTES

RECOMMENDED STORAGE: Storage is not recommended.

Avocado is rich in fatty acids, potassium, and vitamin E, making it incredible for healing dry, irritated, and flaky skin. It helps your skin retain moisture and elasticity, making it great for antiaging. Cacao is full of nutrients that promote blood flow and collagen production, giving you a healthy glow. It also helps protect and repair damaged skin. This is one of my favorite masks to achieve bright and glowing skin. I often use it the night before an event to exfoliate and prepare my skin for the next day.

½ avocado, peeled and pitted

2 tablespoons apple cider vinegar

1 tablespoon raw honey

1 tablespoon cacao powder

1. Put the avocado, apple cider vinegar, raw honey, and cacao powder in a small bowl.

2. Mash the avocado with a fork and mix the ingredients until fully combined.

3. Using a facial brush or your fingers, apply the mask to your face, avoiding your eyes.

4. Lie down and let the mask sit for 15 to 20 minutes.

5. Rinse off the mask with lukewarm water and pat your skin dry with a towel.

6. Follow with a non-pore-clogging moisturizer.

USAGE TIP: The antioxidants in avocado are great for treating sunburn. Try this mask after a day in the sun to heal and soothe your skin.

CUCUMBER MAKEUP-SETTING SPRAY

YIELD: 8 OUNCES | PREP TIME: 2 MINUTES

RECOMMENDED STORAGE: Store in a glass spray bottle.

Cucumber seed essential oil is rich in phytosterols, tocopherols, tocotrienols, and fatty acids, making it a powerhouse antiaging ingredient. It moisturizes the skin while reducing inflammation and redness and encourages skin cell regeneration. This is the perfect spray to set your makeup and hydrate your skin. I use it both pre- and post-makeup application for extra hydration and glow.

1 cup distilled water

2 tablespoons apple cider vinegar

1 tablespoon witch hazel

3 to 4 drops cucumber seed essential oil

1. Put the distilled water, apple cider vinegar, witch hazel, and cucumber seed essential oil in a small bottle. Cover and shake well to combine.

2. After you have applied your makeup, hold the bottle a few inches away from your face and mist your face with one to two pumps. Let air-dry.

USAGE TIP: Use this spray to make your liquid foundation application smoother and provide an extra dose of hydration.

ROSE WATER HYDRATING SKIN SPRITZ

YIELD: 8 OUNCES | PREP TIME: 2 MINUTES

RECOMMENDED STORAGE: Store in a glass spray bottle.

Rose water has been used for thousands of years and is known as "beauty's magic potion." It helps hydrate and revitalize the skin while controlling excess oil. Rose water contains antioxidants that help strengthen and regenerate skin tissues, resulting in glowing, smooth skin. Both the smell and feel are so soothing and relaxing that when you need a skin pick-me-up, this will be your go-to spritz.

½ cup rose water

½ cup distilled water

2 tablespoons apple cider vinegar

3 to 4 drops lavender essential oil

1. Put the rose water, distilled water, apple cider vinegar, and lavender essential oil in a reusable spray bottle. Cover and shake well to combine.

2. Spray on skin any time of day as needed.

VARIATION TIP: For a decorative touch, add 4 or 5 fresh rose petals to the glass spray bottle before filling it with the ingredients.

HEALING CARROT SEED SERUM

YIELD: 2.5 OUNCES | PREP TIME: 2 MINUTES

RECOMMENDED STORAGE: Store in a glass bottle with dropper.

Carrot seed essential oil is wonderful for healing dry, chapped, and cracked skin because it stimulates the growth of new cells and tissues. It contains antioxidants, beta carotene, vitamin A, and vitamin E. Carrot seed essential oil is also great for lightening pigmentation, soothing sunburn, and smoothing wrinkles. This serum is incredibly nourishing. When your skin is dry, it will soak this serum right up. I love to put this on at night so that I wake up with refreshed skin.

4 tablespoons aloe vera gel

1 tablespoon apple cider vinegar

2 teaspoons hemp seed oil

5 drops carrot seed essential oil

1. Put the aloe vera, apple cider vinegar, hemp seed oil, and carrot seed essential oil in a reusable dropper bottle. Cover and shake well to combine.

2. After cleansing your face, rub 4 to 5 drops together in your hands and gently massage onto your face.

HEALTH TIP: Pregnant women should avoid carrot seed essential oil since research has not been conducted to reveal which attributes are passed to the fetus. If your doctor approves, a pregnancy-safe alternative would be ylang-ylang or chamomile essential oil.

OATMEAL-HONEY BATH SOAK

YIELD: 1 TREATMENT | PREP TIME: 10 MINUTES

RECOMMENDED STORAGE: Storage is not recommended.

Oatmeal is very nourishing to the skin. It soothes irritation, reduces inflammation, and relieves itchiness. It also helps rehydrate the skin, leaving it silky, smooth, and calm. With the addition of raw honey's antibacterial and healing properties, this bath soak provides relief from both eczema and mild rashes.

½ cup oats

⅓ cup apple cider vinegar

⅓ cup Epsom salt

4 tablespoons raw honey

1. Put the oats in a blender or food processor, and blend until they become a fine powder. (This step helps the mixture wash down the drain after your bath.)
2. After drawing a warm bath, add the ground oats, apple cider vinegar, Epsom salt, and raw honey to the water.
3. Give everything a big swirl in the tub to mix.
4. Soak in the bath for at least 20 minutes for best results.

VARIATION TIP: Add lavender essential oil for an even more relaxing experience.

HEALTH TIP: Practice slow and relaxed breathing while in the bath to lower stress levels.

MAGNESIUM-SALT SPRAY

**YIELD: 8 OUNCES | PREP TIME: 2 MINUTES | COOK TIME: 10 MINUTES
COOLING TIME: 10 MINUTES**

RECOMMENDED STORAGE: Store in a glass spray bottle.

Sea salt has long been used for therapeutic purposes. The minerals in sea salt nourish and hydrate skin, while also gently removing dead skin cells. It has been used in remedies for years to provide relief and healing for skin conditions, including eczema and psoriasis.

1 cup distilled water

1 tablespoon Himalayan salt or sea salt

¼ teaspoon magnesium flakes

2 tablespoons apple cider vinegar

1. Warm the water in a saucepan on the stove over low heat.

2. Add the salt and magnesium and stir with a spoon until completely dissolved.

3. Remove the mixture from heat and let cool for about 10 minutes (or put it in the refrigerator for 3 to 5 minutes).

4. Once cooled, add the apple cider vinegar and stir to combine.

5. Pour the mixture into a spray bottle and mist all over the body or on irritated areas.

VARIATION TIP: Add any essential oils to this spray. Lavender or peppermint are two great choices specifically for easing eczema.

SIMPLE GREEN ALKALINE SMOOTHIE

YIELD: 1 (20-OUNCE) SERVING | PREP TIME: 10 MINUTES

RECOMMENDED STORAGE: Storage is not recommended.

With eczema, it is just as important to be mindful of what you are putting in your body as what you are putting on it. When your body is too acidic or too low in alkalinity, it can cause additional eczema flare-ups, so it is important to incorporate alkaline foods in your diet. Make this smoothie a staple in your morning routine to help fuel your body and control eczema flare-ups.

1 cup water

1 cup spinach

½ frozen banana

¼ cup frozen riced cauliflower

¼ cup frozen blueberries

2 tablespoons apple cider vinegar

1. Put the water, spinach, banana, cauliflower, blueberries, and apple cider vinegar in a blender. Blend until smooth.

2. If the consistency is too thick, add more water a splash at a time until the consistency is right.

VARIATION TIP: Substitute almond milk or coconut milk for water for a creamier texture.

TEA TREE AND CLOVE ANTIFUNGAL FOOT SOAK

YIELD: 1 TREATMENT | PREP TIME: 5 MINUTES

RECOMMENDED STORAGE: Storage is not recommended.

SPECIAL MATERIALS NEEDED: Bucket or pan deep enough to fully submerge feet.

Apple cider vinegar is a wonderful remedy for foot fungus, toenail fungus, and athlete's foot because it helps disinfect the foot while eliminating odors. Not only does this soak treat fungus, but it also rids your feet of calluses by exfoliating dead skin cells. This is the perfect soak to prepare your feet for summer or give them some much-needed attention in the winter. If you are experiencing an infection, soak daily until the infection subsides. You can gradually increase the time you soak over several weeks to up to 30 minutes.

1 gallon very warm water

2 cups apple cider vinegar

½ cup Epsom salt

15 drops lavender essential oil

1. Fill the bucket or pan with very warm water.

2. Add the apple cider vinegar, Epsom salt, and lavender essential oil.

3. Put your feet in the mixture and let soak for 10 to 15 minutes.

HEALTH TIP: If you are struggling with athlete's foot or foot fungus, remember to wear breathable socks and give your feet a break from close-toed shoes by going barefoot at home or wearing sandals while you are out.

ATHLETE'S FOOT PROBIOTIC SALVE

**YIELD: ABOUT 57 (TEASPOON-SIZE) APPLICATIONS | PREP TIME: 2 MINUTES
COOK TIME: 10 MINUTES**

RECOMMENDED STORAGE: Store in a tin or glass jar.

When the skin's bacteria are unbalanced or the skin lacks beneficial bacteria, fungal infections have the opportunity to form. When this happens, it is necessary to bring the skin's bacteria back to balance. Probiotics containing *saccharomyces boulardii* provide a beneficial antifungal yeast that can help your skin fight and heal fungal infections.

1 cup shea butter

3 tablespoons apple cider vinegar

40 drops tea tree essential oil

10 drops oregano essential oil

3 probiotic capsules containing *saccharomyces boulardii*

1. Heat the shea butter in a double boiler (or a large glass or metal bowl set over a pot of boiling water) until melted.

2. Remove from heat and add the apple cider vinegar, tea tree essential oil, oregano essential oil. Open probiotic capsules and pour the contents into the mixture with other ingredients. Stir with a spoon until fully mixed.

3. Pour the mixture into a reusable jar or tin.

4. Apply a teaspoon-size amount to the infected area as often as needed when the feeling of itching and stinging comes on or your feet begin to get dry and cracked.

USAGE TIP: Although the butter will take several hours to set, it can also be used as a liquid. This butter can also be used as a supermoisturizing hand lotion to soothe cracked and dry skin.

SOOTHING PEPPERMINT FOOT SCRUB

YIELD: APPROXIMATELY 14 OUNCES, OR 42 (TEASPOON-SIZE) APPLICATIONS
PREP TIME: 5 MINUTES

RECOMMENDED STORAGE: Store in an airtight glass jar.

Epsom salt is very different from table salt. It is a magnesium sulfate compound packed full of nutrients. The magnesium in Epsom salt can increase magnesium levels in the body to reduce swelling, eliminate odor, and help treat infections. It can also be an effective pain reliever. This foot scrub removes dead skin cells, cleanses the skin, and works to get rid of any foot bacteria or fungus. It will also hydrate your skin and soothe irritation.

1 cup Epsom salt

½ cup almond oil

4 tablespoons apple cider vinegar

10 to 15 drops peppermint essential oil

1. Put the Epsom salt, almond oil, apple cider vinegar, and peppermint essential oil in a glass jar. Stir until fully mixed.

2. While feet are wet, apply a teaspoon-size amount to each foot and scrub for about 30 seconds. Rinse with warm water.

USAGE TIP: This scrub can be used once a week to keep skin smooth or several times per week if needed. You can also use this scrub for a full-body exfoliation (excluding the face) to remove dead skin cells and leave your skin smooth and hydrated.

EUCALYPTUS HAND-REPAIR CREAM

YIELD: 8 OUNCES, OR 48 (TEASPOON-SIZE) APPLICATIONS
PREP TIME: 2 MINUTES | COOK TIME: 10 MINUTES

RECOMMENDED STORAGE: Store in a tin or glass jar.

Apple cider vinegar helps balance the skin's pH, resulting in healing and regeneration. Honey helps prevent free-radical damage, nourishes the skin, and is a natural antibacterial. This hand cream is rich in antioxidants, amino acids, vitamins, and enzymes from the raw honey. It's one of my favorites, especially in the winter when hands can get extra dry. Your silky smooth hands will thank you.

½ cup shea butter

¼ cup almond oil

3 tablespoons apple cider vinegar

2 tablespoons raw honey

40 drops eucalyptus essential oil

1. Heat the shea butter in a double boiler (or a large glass or metal bowl set over a pot of simmering water) until melted.

2. Remove from heat and add the almond oil, apple cider vinegar, raw honey, and eucalyptus essential oil. Stir until fully mixed.

3. Pour the mixture into reusable jar.

4. Massage a teaspoon-size amount into your hands until fully absorbed.

USAGE TIP: Although the cream will take several hours to fully set, it can also be used as a liquid.

BRITTLE NAIL RECOVERY TREATMENT

YIELD: 1 TREATMENT | PREP TIME: 2 MINUTES

RECOMMENDED STORAGE: Storage is not recommended.

Over time, consistently having acrylic nails or using gel polish, or even regular nail polish, breaks down the strength and quality of your nails. This treatment helps restore and increase the health of your nails. Apple cider vinegar contains calcium, iron, potassium, and magnesium to improve the strength of your nails. Lavender essential oil works to reverse weak and brittle nails, as well as providing antibacterial properties. This is my favorite recovery treatment after removing a gel manicure because it helps keep my nails strong and thick.

¼ cup warm water

¼ cup apple cider vinegar

5 drops lavender essential oil

1. In a small bowl, combine the warm water, apple cider vinegar, and lavender essential oil.
2. Soak your fingertips for at least 5 minutes, then rinse with water and pat your hands dry with a towel.
3. Apply a deep moisturizing cream such as the Eucalyptus Hand-Repair Cream (page 81) to your hands as the perfect follow-up.

USAGE TIP: Use weekly for best results.

PUMPKIN PIE HAND SCRUB

YIELD: 6 OUNCES, OR 36 (TEASPOON-SIZE) APPLICATIONS | PREP TIME: 5 MINUTES

RECOMMENDED STORAGE: Store in a sealed glass jar.

You use your hands every single day, so why not give them a boost? This scrub dissolves dead skin cells and reveals healthy, glowing skin. Hemp seed oil is highly moisturizing and leaves the skin feeling silky smooth. It is also an anti-inflammatory and antibacterial and contains antioxidants that protect against premature aging. Cinnamon helps increase blood circulation and can help alleviate ringworm, eczema, and other skin infections.

½ cup brown sugar

¼ cup hemp seed oil

2 tablespoons apple cider vinegar

1 teaspoon raw honey

3 to 5 drops cinnamon essential oil

½ teaspoon pumpkin pie spice

1. Put the brown sugar, hemp seed oil, apple cider vinegar, raw honey, cinnamon essential oil, and pumpkin pie spice in a bowl and mix with a spoon until well combined.

2. Pour the mixture into a sealable glass jar.

3. To apply, scoop out 1 teaspoon of the mixture and massage into wet hands, making sure to lightly scrub your cuticles as well.

4. Rinse your hands and follow with a moisturizing lotion, such as the Eucalyptus Hand-Repair Cream (page 81).

INGREDIENT TIP: Make sure to use a 100 percent unrefined hemp seed oil to avoid filler agents that could lead to irritation. Refined hemp seed oil also lacks the many benefits that the unrefined version contains.

LEMON-SANDALWOOD TONER

YIELD: 8 OUNCES | PREP TIME: 2 MINUTES

RECOMMENDED STORAGE: Store in a glass bottle.

Apple cider vinegar works to balance the skin's pH, making skin less dry and killing bacteria. Lemon essential oil has natural brightening and antifungal properties, which makes it great for reducing hyperpigmentation and killing acne-causing bacteria. Sandalwood essential oil, a natural anti-inflammatory, helps reduce the inflammation caused by acne, scrapes, and rashes. Sandalwood is also a natural skin lightener and helps even skin tone. When I am trying to quickly heal pigmentation left over from breakouts, this is my go-to toner for speeding up the healing process.

1 cup distilled water

2 tablespoons apple cider vinegar

10 drops lemon essential oil

4 drops sandalwood essential oil

1. Put the water, apple cider vinegar, lemon essential oil, and sandalwood essential oil in a reusable glass bottle. Seal the bottle and shake well to combine.

2. Pour a small amount onto a cotton pad and gently apply to your skin after cleansing. Be sure to avoid your eyes.

PINEAPPLE ENZYME MASK

YIELD: 1 TREATMENT | PREP TIME: 5 MINUTES

RECOMMENDED STORAGE: Storage is not recommended.

Pineapple contains a large amount of the enzyme bromelain, which removes the dead outer layers of the skin, reduces inflammation, and brightens the skin for an ultimate glow. It also contains the powerhouse ingredient vitamin C, which helps repair sun-damaged skin and uneven skin tone. When my skin looks a little dull, I turn to this mask for an intense brightening and fresh skin.

½ cup fresh pineapple

2 tablespoons apple cider vinegar

1 teaspoon raw honey

1. Put the pineapple, apple cider vinegar, and raw honey in a blender. Blend until smooth.

2. After cleansing your skin, use a facial brush or your fingers to gently apply the mask to your face, avoiding your eyes.

3. Lie down and let the mask sit for 5 to 10 minutes. You will feel some light tingling, which is the enzymes doing their work.

4. Rinse off your mask with lukewarm water and pat your skin dry with a towel.

5. Follow with a non-pore-clogging moisturizer.

HEALTH TIP: Pineapple is very acidic, which can cause a skin reaction for some people. Test a piece of pineapple on the inside of your wrist. If there is any irritation within 1 to 3 hours, do not use pineapple on your skin.

APPLE PIE BRIGHTENING SKIN MASK

YIELD: 1 TREATMENT | PREP TIME: 2 MINUTES

RECOMMENDED STORAGE: Storage is not recommended.

This apple and honey combination is a super source of vitamins and nutrients for your skin. Applesauce and apple cider vinegar contain acids that work to gently dissolve dead skin cells and clarify your skin. Honey delivers a host of vitamins and amino acids, giving you a hydrated, soft glow, while cinnamon increases blood flow and fights acne. This mask can be used weekly for an exfoliating, nutrient-dense skin boost.

2 tablespoons applesauce (no additives and preferably organic)

2 tablespoons apple cider vinegar

1 tablespoon raw honey

2 dashes cinnamon

1. In a small bowl, combine the applesauce, apple cider vinegar, raw honey, and cinnamon.
2. After cleansing your skin, use a facial brush or your fingers to gently apply the mask to your face, avoiding your eyes.
3. Lie down and let the mask sit for 10 to 15 minutes. You may feel some light tingling.
4. Rinse off your mask with lukewarm water and pat your skin dry with a towel.
5. Follow with a non-pore-clogging moisturizer.

LAVENDER-LEMON INGROWN-HAIR SPRAY

YIELD: 8 OUNCES | PREP TIME: 2 MINUTES

RECOMMENDED STORAGE: Store in a glass spray bottle.

The combination of apple cider vinegar and witch hazel makes a powerful anti-inflammatory and helps reduce redness. It also helps exfoliate dead skin cells and fight the bacteria that can lead to infected ingrown hairs. Tea tree essential oil and lemon essential oil work to tighten pores and kill bacteria. Lavender essential oil helps soothe and calm irritated, itchy skin. This spray is great to apply after shaving as well as before exercising because sweating can increase your chances of ingrown hairs.

1 cup distilled water

2 tablespoons apple cider vinegar

2 tablespoons witch hazel

4 to 5 drops lavender essential oil

4 to 5 drops lemon essential oil

4 to 5 drops tea tree essential oil

1. In a glass spray bottle, combine the water, apple cider vinegar, witch hazel, lavender essential oil, lemon essential oil, and tea tree essential oil. Seal the bottle and shake to combine.

2. To apply, mist over irritated areas, as well as areas prone to ingrown hairs, and let air-dry.

INGROWN HAIR–FIGHTING SUGAR SCRUB

YIELD: 14 OUNCES, OR 84 (TEASPOON-SIZE) APPLICATIONS | PREP TIME: 5 MINUTES

RECOMMENDED STORAGE: Store in an airtight glass jar.

Sugar makes an amazing exfoliant that is safe even for people with sensitive skin. It works to remove dead skin cells, making it easier for ingrown hairs to be released. Jojoba oil hydrates and nourishes the newly exfoliated skin, and tea tree essential oil has antibacterial and antiseptic properties that help fight infections while also providing relief and reducing redness. The best way to take action is to prevent ingrown hairs from occurring in the first place. Use this scrub weekly in the areas prone to ingrown hairs.

1 cup granulated sugar

½ cup jojoba oil

4 tablespoons apple cider vinegar

10 drops tea tree essential oil

1. In a sealable glass jar, stir together the sugar, jojoba oil, apple cider vinegar, and tea tree essential oil until fully combined.

2. Apply a teaspoon-size amount to wet skin in the affected area and gently exfoliate for about 30 seconds.

3. Rinse, pat dry, and apply a non-pore-clogging moisturizer.

VARIATION TIP: If you have extra jojoba oil, it is a perfect moisturizer to apply to areas prone to ingrown hairs.

PEPPERMINT-VANILLA LIP SCRUB

YIELD: 8 OUNCES, OR 48 (½-TEASPOON-SIZE) APPLICATIONS | PREP TIME: 5 MINUTES

RECOMMENDED STORAGE: Store in an airtight glass jar.

A proper exfoliant should remove dead skin cells and hydrate. Sugar makes a great exfoliant that is gentle enough not to cause damage to your skin. Hemp seed oil contains essential fatty acids and omega 3, 6, and 9, which all help hydrate your lips. Peppermint provides a cooling effect, giving your lips a refreshed feeling. I use this scrub on a weekly basis to keep my lips healthy and hydrated and to allow moisturizing lip balm to do its work even more effectively.

¼ cup granulated sugar

2 tablespoons apple cider vinegar

2 tablespoons hemp seed oil

2 to 4 drops peppermint essential oil

10 drops vanilla essential oil

1. In a small bowl combine the sugar, apple cider vinegar, hemp seed oil, peppermint essential oil, and vanilla essential oil. (Peppermint is very strong. Start with 2 drops and add as you try the mixture.)

2. Stir until fully mixed.

3. Store in an airtight jar.

4. When you are ready to use, take a small amount (about ½ teaspoon) and rub gently on your lips for about 30 seconds.

5. Let the scrub sit for 2 minutes, then remove with a warm washcloth, gently exfoliating as you remove it.

6. Follow with a moisturizing lip balm.

GRAPEFRUIT-THYME UNDERARM DETOX TREATMENT

YIELD: 8 OUNCES | PREP TIME: 2 MINUTES

RECOMMENDED STORAGE: Store in a glass spray bottle.

When switching from conventional to natural deodorant, you should give your underarms a little detox and restart. This can help your body get back to its natural state of detoxing by flushing out old bacterial and chemical residue. Apple cider vinegar helps balance the body's pH level and stimulates detoxification, while the essential oils provide antibacterial and antifungal benefits.

3 tablespoons apple cider vinegar

4 to 5 drops grapefruit essential oil

4 to 5 drops thyme essential oil

1 cup water

1. Put the apple cider vinegar, grapefruit essential oil, and thyme essential oil in a glass spray bottle.

2. Top off the bottle with water. (You may not need the full amount.) Cover and shake well to combine.

3. Shake well before each use. Spray both underarms.

4. Let air-dry.

USAGE TIP: This treatment is best used at night when you are not wearing any deodorant, whether conventional or natural.

GERANIUM-CYPRESS VARICOSE VEIN SPRAY

YIELD: 8 OUNCES | PREP TIME: 2 MINUTES

RECOMMENDED STORAGE: Store in a glass spray bottle.

When it comes to varicose veins, cypress is the holy grail of essential oils because it supports the circulatory system by encouraging blood to flow properly. Geranium stimulates blood circulation, while also treating the appearance of varicose veins. Together with apple cider vinegar, these ingredients alleviate the symptoms and appearance of varicose veins. This spray also works well for reducing the visibility of stretch marks and can be used multiple times a day.

4 tablespoons apple cider vinegar

5 to 7 drops cypress essential oil

5 to 7 drops geranium essential oil

1 cup distilled water

1. Pour the apple cider vinegar, cypress essential oil, and geranium essential oil into a glass spray bottle. Top off the bottle with water. (You may not need the full amount.) Seal the bottle and shake to combine.

2. To apply, mist over varicose veins while massaging the area.

LEMON-GINGER VARICOSE VEIN MASSAGE OIL

YIELD: 8 OUNCES | PREP TIME: 2 MINUTES

RECOMMENDED STORAGE: Store in a glass bottle.

Stimulating blood circulation is key when you have varicose veins, and lemon essential oil does just that. It also provides an uplifting but calming effect. Ginger essential oil has both anesthetic and anti-inflammatory properties that help reduce aching and discomfort.

1 cup jojoba oil

3 tablespoons apple cider vinegar

10 to 12 drops lemon essential oil

10 to 12 drops ginger essential oil

1. In a reusable glass bottle, combine the jojoba oil, apple cider vinegar, lemon essential oil, and ginger essential oil. Shake well to combine.

2. To apply, pour a quarter-size amount into your hands and massage into the areas where varicose veins are present for 5 to 10 minutes.

CHAMOMILE-SAGE VARICOSE VEIN BATH SOAK

YIELD: 1 TREATMENT | PREP TIME: 10 MINUTES

RECOMMENDED STORAGE: Storage is not recommended.

Chamomile has anti-inflammatory and antioxidant effects that can help reduce the discomfort of varicose veins. Clary sage can be extremely beneficial for people with varicose veins; many people have trouble sleeping due to the aching and discomfort, and clary sage oil creates a calming effect to improve sleep quality and reduce blood pressure. Combining these in a warm bath can increase blood flow and provide major relief.

½ cup Epsom salt

⅓ cup apple cider vinegar

10 to 15 drops chamomile essential oil

5 to 7 drops clary sage essential oil

1. Draw a warm bath and add the Epsom salt, apple cider vinegar, chamomile essential oil, and clary sage essential oil.

2. Give everything a big swirl with your hands in the tub to mix.

3. Soak in the bath for at least 20 minutes for best results.

USAGE TIP: After your bath, massage Lemon-Ginger Varicose Vein Massage Oil (page 92) into your skin for the ultimate healing effect.

LAVENDER-OATMEAL SUNBURN SOAK

YIELD: 1 TREATMENT | PREP TIME: 10 MINUTES

RECOMMENDED STORAGE: Storage is not recommended.

Oatmeal is a star ingredient when treating sunburn because it helps soothe, moisturize, and promote skin repair. It can also help reduce that burning sensation that comes along with sunburn. Lavender essential oil helps speed up the healing and recovery process because it also has anti-inflammatory properties that aid in burn relief. Additionally, apple cider vinegar contains cooling and calming properties that make it the perfect sunburn remedy.

½ cup oats

⅓ cup apple cider vinegar

10 to 12 drops lavender essential oil

1. Put the oats in a blender or food processor. Blend until they are a fine powder. (This step helps the mixture wash down the drain after your bath.)

2. Draw a warm bath to your ideal temperature. If you are severely sunburned, you may want to go with a bath on the cooler or lukewarm side.

3. Add the oats, apple cider vinegar, and lavender essential oil to the bath.

4. Give everything a big swirl with your hands in the tub to mix.

5. Soak in the bath for at least 20 minutes for best results.

SUNBURN HEALING SPRAY

YIELD: 8 OUNCES | PREP TIME: 2 MINUTES

RECOMMENDED STORAGE: Store in a glass spray bottle.

Sunburns are no fun. I remember going to the beach every summer and always returning with a sunburn. I have used this recipe for years to rapidly heal my skin and provide relief. Calendula is known as one of nature's most healing herbs. It is rich in antioxidants and both nourishes and soothes sunburned skin. Geranium essential oil relieves pain caused by burned skin and is an anti-inflammatory. Lavender and chamomile increase wound healing and reduce redness. Sandalwood has cooling properties, helping to take away that painful heat.

½ cup distilled water

¼ cup calendula oil

2 tablespoons apple cider vinegar

5 to 7 drops geranium essential oil

5 to 7 drops lavender essential oil

5 to 7 drops chamomile essential oil

5 to 7 drops sandalwood essential oil

1. Put the water, calendula oil, apple cider vinegar, geranium essential oil, lavender essential oil, chamomile essential oil, and sandalwood essential oil in a glass spray bottle. Shake well to combine.

2. To apply, mist over entire body, or over sunburned areas.

USAGE TIP: Use this mixture throughout the day as needed.

HYDRATING SUNBURN TONIC

YIELD: 2 (8-OUNCE) SERVINGS | PREP TIME: 10 MINUTES

RECOMMENDED STORAGE: You can store the watermelon mixture (without the sparkling water added) in a sealed glass jar for up to 24 hours in the refrigerator.

When you get sunburned, your body temperature rises, in turn dehydrating you. In addition to avoiding sun exposure and topically treating your sunburn, it is vital to stay hydrated so that your body can heal faster and more efficiently. Watermelon contains important vitamins and electrolytes that help hydrate your body more than water alone can. This tonic is a delicious and refreshing way to hydrate your body and heal from sunburn.

1 cup cubed watermelon

¼ cup sliced cucumber

2 tablespoons apple cider vinegar

2 to 3 mint leaves

½ cup sparkling water

1. Put the watermelon, cucumber, apple cider vinegar, and mint leaves in a blender. Blend until smooth.

2. Divide the watermelon mixture evenly into two glasses and top off with the sparkling water. (You may not need the full amount.) Sip and enjoy.

Hair

Whether your hair is long or short, curly or straight, healthy hair is indispensable. Though we clean our hair regularly, scalp care is an often-overlooked but essential step of hair care. This section provides simple, natural recipes to tackle dandruff, dry and dull hair, oily hair, lice, and hair growth.

FEATURED RECIPES: Peppermint-Aloe Hair Rinse (98), Green Tea and Salt Scalp Scrub (99), Nourishing Rosemary Hair Mask (100), Lavender-Avocado Hair Treatment (101), Argan-Citrus Essential Hair Oil (102), Ylang-Ylang Hydration Boost Rinse (103), Calming Chamomile-Salt Scalp Scrub (104), Lavender-Lemon Scalp Cleanser (105), Tea Tree Hair Mask (106), Coconut Oil–Tea Tree Lice Treatment (107), Rosemary-Thyme-Salt Scalp Scrub (108), Healthy Hair Elixir (109), Nettle Hair-Growth Tea (110) and Lavender Hair Therapy (111).

PEPPERMINT-ALOE HAIR RINSE

YIELD: 1 TREATMENT | PREP TIME: 2 MINUTES

RECOMMENDED STORAGE: Storage is not recommended.

Apple cider vinegar works to balance the pH of your hair. It gently cleanses without stripping the hair of natural oils or color. It soothes, calms, and exfoliates the scalp while providing hydration. Peppermint essential oil helps with dandruff because of its anti-inflammatory and antiseptic properties. It also stimulates hair growth and helps strengthen hair roots.

½ cup distilled water

½ cup apple cider vinegar

¼ cup aloe vera water

2 drops peppermint essential oil

1. Put the water, apple cider vinegar, aloe vera water, and peppermint essential oil in a large cup and mix together with a spoon.

2. Wet your scalp and hair and squeeze out excess water.

3. Massage the mixture into your scalp, creating small parts in your hair to work it in deeply.

4. Let the mixture sit for 2 to 3 minutes and rinse thoroughly.

GREEN TEA AND SALT SCALP SCRUB

YIELD: 13 OUNCES, OR 26 (TABLESPOON-SIZE) APPLICATIONS | PREP TIME: 5 MINUTES

RECOMMENDED STORAGE: Store in a glass jar.

Pink Himalayan salt naturally removes product buildup, dead skin cells, and impurities. Avocado oil and green tea provide a soothing, hydrating effect, and apple cider vinegar rebalances hair's pH levels and soothes irritated scalps. This scrub is perfect for dry, oily, or combination hair.

1 cup pink Himalayan salt (fine crystals)

¼ cup avocado oil

¼ cup brewed and cooled green tea

3 tablespoons apple cider vinegar

1. Put the Himalayan sea salt, avocado oil, green tea, and apple cider vinegar in a glass jar and mix thoroughly with a spoon.

2. Wet your scalp and hair and squeeze out excess water.

3. Massage about 1 tablespoon of the scrub into your scalp for 1 to 2 minutes, working from your hairline all the way to the back of your head. Do not pull the scrub through your hair.

4. Rinse the scrub fully out of your hair. If you have long hair, you may want to flip your head over to rinse.

VARIATION TIP: Substitute olive oil or hemp seed oil for the avocado oil.

NOURISHING ROSEMARY HAIR MASK

YIELD: 4 OUNCES | PREP TIME: 2 MINUTES

RECOMMENDED STORAGE: Store in a glass spray bottle.

Apple cider vinegar works to unclog your hair follicles and cleanse your scalp to provide relief from dandruff; rosemary essential oil has antiseptic and antimicrobial properties that help eliminate it. Dandruff is caused by an overgrowth of yeast, which rosemary's antifungal properties help kill. It also soothes the itchy scalp that comes along with dandruff.

¼ cup water

¼ cup apple cider vinegar

5 to 7 drops rosemary essential oil

1. In a glass spray bottle, combine the water, apple cider vinegar, and rosemary essential oil and shake well to combine.

2. Spray the solution all over your hair and scalp.

3. Let it sit for at least 15 minutes before rinsing it out.

USAGE TIP: This mask works best after the Green Tea and Salt Scalp Scrub (page 99) is used.

LAVENDER-AVOCADO HAIR TREATMENT

YIELD: 4 OUNCES | PREP TIME: 2 MINUTES

RECOMMENDED STORAGE: Store in a glass dropper bottle.

Many hair products dry hair out, leaving it with a dull look and feel. Used before shampooing, this treatment will smooth, soften, and condition your hair for an extra boost of shine and hydration. Avocado oil is one of the only oils that can penetrate the hair shaft and moisturize your hair. It contains healthy acids and fats that strengthen, heal, and prevent further damage. Lavender essential oil deeply conditions hair and helps keep it shiny. This is my favorite treatment because it leaves my hair feeling smooth and shiny and even helps my hair last longer in between washes.

2 tablespoons avocado oil

2 tablespoons apple cider vinegar

5 to 7 drops lavender essential oil

1. In a glass dropper bottle, combine the avocado oil, apple cider vinegar, and lavender essential oil and shake well to combine.

2. Squeeze 5 to 7 drops of treatment into your hand and massage into your scalp, pulling through to the ends of your hair. Depending on how much hair you have, you may need more.

3. Let sit at least 15 minutes before shampooing and conditioning as normal.

USAGE TIP: Use a pea-size amount of this treatment on the ends of dry hair to prevent split ends and heal damage.

ARGAN-CITRUS ESSENTIAL HAIR OIL

YIELD: 4 OUNCES | PREP TIME: 2 MINUTES

RECOMMENDED STORAGE: Store in a glass dropper bottle.

Argan oil is a beauty secret that has been used for centuries to bring life back into hair. The essential fatty acids, antioxidants, and vitamins in argan oil provide deep hydration and nutrients, resulting in soft, shiny, hydrated hair. It also helps protect your hair from free radicals that lead to splitting and breakage. Lemon and grapefruit essential oils provide extra conditioning and shine support. I love the smell of this oil! My hair feels so nourished and smooth after using it.

2 tablespoons argan oil

2 tablespoons apple cider vinegar

4 to 5 drops lemon essential oil

4 to 5 drops grapefruit essential oil

1. Put the argan oil, apple cider vinegar, lemon essential oil, and grapefruit oil in a reusable dropper bottle. Shake well to combine.

2. After drying and styling your hair, squeeze 5 to 7 drops into your hand and run it through your hair from the back of your head to your hairline, pulling it through to the ends of your hair.

YLANG-YLANG HYDRATION BOOST RINSE

YIELD: 1 TREATMENT | PREP TIME: 2 MINUTES

Aloe vera contains powerful enzymes that repair skin cells on the scalp. Its vitamins and nutrients keep your scalp and hair moisturized and conditioned for ultimate shine. Ylang-ylang essential oil serves as a natural conditioner by stimulating the production of sebum (oil) in your hair. It also helps prevent damage and split ends.

½ cup distilled water

½ cup apple cider vinegar

¼ cup aloe vera water

5 to 7 drops ylang-ylang essential oil

1. Put the water, apple cider vinegar, aloe vera water, and ylang-ylang essential oil in a large cup and stir to combine.
2. Wet your scalp and hair and squeeze out excess water.
3. Slowly massage the mixture into your scalp, creating small parts in your hair to work it in deeply.
4. Leave on for 2 to 3 minutes and then rinse thoroughly.

CALMING CHAMOMILE-SALT SCALP SCRUB

YIELD: 13 OUNCES, OR 26 (TABLESPOON-SIZE) APPLICATIONS | PREP TIME: 5 MINUTES

RECOMMENDED STORAGE: Store in a glass jar.

Hair can begin to look dull and lifeless when a surplus of products builds up on the scalp, because the buildup hinders the natural production of the oils that give your hair a healthy shine. Himalayan salt works to remove dead skin cells and product buildup so that oils can be freely produced and hair products can work correctly. Avocado oil is the ultimate hair moisturizer, delivering a deep conditioning. Chamomile tea fights against dandruff, nourishes your hair, and helps prevent split ends.

1 cup pink Himalayan salt (fine crystals)

¼ cup avocado oil

¼ cup brewed and cooled chamomile tea

3 tablespoons apple cider vinegar

1. Put the pink Himalayan salt, avocado oil, chamomile tea, and apple cider vinegar in a bowl and mix thoroughly with a spoon. Transfer the mixture to a glass jar.

2. Wet your scalp and hair and squeeze out excess water.

3. Massage about 1 tablespoon of the scrub into your scalp for 1 to 2 minutes, working from your hairline all the way to the back of your head. Do not pull through your hair.

4. Rinse the scrub out of your hair completely. If you have long hair, you may want to flip your head over to rinse.

VARIATION TIP: Substitute olive oil or hemp seed oil for the avocado oil.

LAVENDER-LEMON SCALP CLEANSER

YIELD: 1 TREATMENT | PREP TIME: 2 MINUTES

RECOMMENDED STORAGE: Storage is not recommended.

Harsh chemicals in hair cleansers can clog your pores and leave a greasy residue on your scalp. By making a homemade cleanser, you can help balance the oil on your scalp and exfoliate to ensure proper oil production. Baking soda and apple cider vinegar help remove product and excess oil buildup while balancing the pH of your scalp. Lavender essential oil improves overall scalp health, and lemon essential oil will help soften and strengthen your hair.

2 tablespoons baking soda

2 tablespoons apple cider vinegar

2 drops lavender essential oil

2 drops lemon essential oil

Splash of water

1. Put the baking soda, apple cider vinegar, lavender essential oil, lemon essential oil, and a splash of water in a small bowl. Mix with a spoon to make a thin paste.

2. Wet your scalp and hair and squeeze out excess water.

3. Using your fingers, massage the mixture onto your wet scalp and leave on for 2 to 3 minutes.

4. Rinse the mixture out of your hair completely.

5. Follow with a conditioner, avoiding the roots of your hair.

TEA TREE HAIR MASK

YIELD: 4 OUNCES | PREP TIME: 5 MINUTES

RECOMMENDED STORAGE: Store in a glass spray bottle.

Clogged pores on your scalp can cause your scalp to overproduce oil. Avocado and honey provide protein, vitamins, and amino acids, which all support healthy hair. Tea tree essential oil clears the excess oil buildup, allowing the pores to breathe and produce oil at normal levels. This mask shows best results when applied weekly until the oil production in your hair is rebalanced.

1 avocado, peeled and pitted

2 tablespoons apple cider vinegar

2 tablespoons raw honey

2 to 3 drops tea tree essential oil

1. Put the avocado, apple cider vinegar, raw honey, and tea tree essential oil in a bowl.
2. Mash the avocado with a fork and mix all ingredients until the consistency is smooth.
3. Wet your scalp and hair and squeeze out excess water.
4. Apply the mask all over your hair and scalp and let it sit for at least 15 minutes before rinsing it out.

USAGE TIP: This mask is best followed by the Lavender-Lemon Scalp Cleanser (page 105).

COCONUT OIL–TEA TREE LICE TREATMENT

YIELD: 1 TREATMENT | PREP TIME: 2 MINUTES

SPECIAL MATERIALS NEEDED: Nit comb

RECOMMENDED STORAGE: Storage is not recommended.

This mask effectively suffocates lice and provides a natural alternative to chemical treatments. The fatty acids found in coconut oil (capric acid, lauric acid, and caprylic acid) make your hair slippery and challenging for lice to move about in, making it easier to comb them out. Coconut oil also helps prevent lice from spreading to clothes and other people. Apple cider vinegar works to dissolve the glue that lice produce in order to stick in your hair, and tea tree essential oil is a natural insecticide that aids in killing lice.

¼ cup coconut oil

¼ cup apple cider vinegar

5 to 7 drops tea tree essential oil

1. Put the coconut oil, apple cider vinegar, and tea tree essential oil in a bowl and mix with a spoon until well combined.

2. Apply the mixture all over your hair and scalp, put on a shower cap, and let sit for 15 to 20 minutes.

3. Remove the shower cap and comb out the lice and eggs with a nit comb.

4. Shampoo and condition your hair as normal.

ROSEMARY-THYME-SALT SCALP SCRUB

YIELD: 11 OUNCES, OR 22 (TABLESPOON-SIZE) APPLICATIONS | PREP TIME: 5 MINUTES

RECOMMENDED STORAGE: Store in a glass jar.

If you are struggling with hair growth, your hair might just need a little reboot. This scrub unclogs pores and clarifies your scalp to allow deep absorption of the essential oils that stimulate hair growth in the follicles. Rosemary essential oil boosts cell regeneration and helps improve the thickness of your hair. Thyme essential oil works to both prevent hair loss and stimulate hair growth. When you combine both oils with the pH balancing of apple cider vinegar and the moisturizing benefits of avocado oil, you have an incredible hair growth scrub.

1 cup pink Himalayan salt (fine crystals)

¼ cup avocado oil

3 tablespoons apple cider vinegar

10 to 12 drops rosemary essential oil

10 to 12 drops thyme essential oil

1. Put the Himalayan salt, avocado oil, apple cider vinegar, rosemary essential oil, and thyme essential oil in a bowl and mix thoroughly. Transfer the mixture to a glass jar.
2. Wet your scalp and hair and squeeze out excess water.
3. Massage about 1 tablespoon of the scrub into your scalp for 1 to 2 minutes, working from your hairline all the way to the back of your head. Do not pull through your hair.
4. Rinse the scrub out of your hair completely. If you have long hair, you may want to flip your head over to rinse.

VARIATION TIP: Substitute olive oil or hemp seed oil for the avocado oil.

HEALTHY HAIR ELIXIR

YIELD: 4 OUNCES | PREP TIME: 2 MINUTES

RECOMMENDED STORAGE: Store in a glass dropper bottle.

Used before shampooing, this treatment will smooth, soften, and condition your hair for an extra boost of shine and hydration. Apple cider vinegar works to balance the pH level of your hair and kill any bacteria that prevents it from being its healthiest. Sunflower seed oil is extremely moisturizing and high in vitamin E and oleic acid, which are responsible for healthy hair growth and the prevention of breakage.

2 tablespoons apple cider vinegar

1 tablespoon avocado oil

1 tablespoon sunflower seed oil

4 to 5 drops clary sage essential oil

4 to 5 drops ylang-ylang essential oil

2 to 3 drops tea tree essential oil

1. In a glass dropper bottle, combine the apple cider vinegar, avocado oil, sunflower seed oil, clary sage essential oil, ylang-ylang essential oil, and tea tree essential oil.

2. Squeeze 5 to 7 drops of treatment into your hand and massage into your scalp, pulling through to the ends of your hair. Depending on how much hair you have, you may need more.

3. Let sit at least 15 minutes before shampooing and conditioning as normal.

USAGE TIP: When your hair is dry, you can also use this as a moisturizing and split-end recovery serum by applying it to the bottom half of your hair, avoiding your roots.

NETTLE HAIR-GROWTH TEA

YIELD: 1 (8-OUNCE) SERVING | PREP TIME: 5 MINUTES | INFUSION TIME: 10 MINUTES

RECOMMENDED STORAGE: Storage is not recommended.

Nettle tea contains vitamins and minerals, such as magnesium, iron, and calcium, and high levels of antioxidants. These play an important role in scalp circulation and hair growth. One of the most interesting aspects of nettle is that it can inhibit the formation of DHT, the hormone that causes baldness. Consuming one to two cups of nettle tea every day can accelerate the growth of healthy, strong hair. When nettle is combined with apple cider vinegar, which helps stimulate blood flow, they work together to promote hair growth.

1 teaspoon dried nettle leaves

1 cup water

2 tablespoons apple cider vinegar

1. Pack the dried nettle leaves in a tea infuser and put in a mug (or add the nettle directly to the mug if you do not have an infuser).

2. Bring the water to a boil and pour it over the tea. Let steep for 10 minutes, then remove the infuser (or strain the tea into a clean mug).

3. Stir the apple cider vinegar into the tea, sip, and enjoy.

LAVENDER HAIR THERAPY

YIELD: 8 OUNCES | PREP TIME: 15 MINUTES

RECOMMENDED STORAGE: Store in a glass spray bottle.

Dandelion tea, argan oil, and aloe leaf juice moisturize and condition your hair without weighing it down. With the addition of lavender essential oil, this spray helps naturally seal the hair's cuticles and rebalance its pH. It is color safe and good for all hair types. After you wash your hair, make this the first step of your post-shower hair routine.

½ cup brewed and cooled dandelion tea

2 tablespoons apple cider vinegar

2 tablespoons argan oil

2 tablespoons aloe leaf juice

20 drops lavender essential oil

¼ cup water

1. In a glass spray bottle, combine the dandelion tea, apple cider vinegar, argan oil, aloe leaf juice, and lavender essential oil. Top off the bottle with water. (You may not need the full amount.) Seal the bottle and shake to combine.

2. Shampoo and condition your hair as normal. Spray on wet hair and comb through.

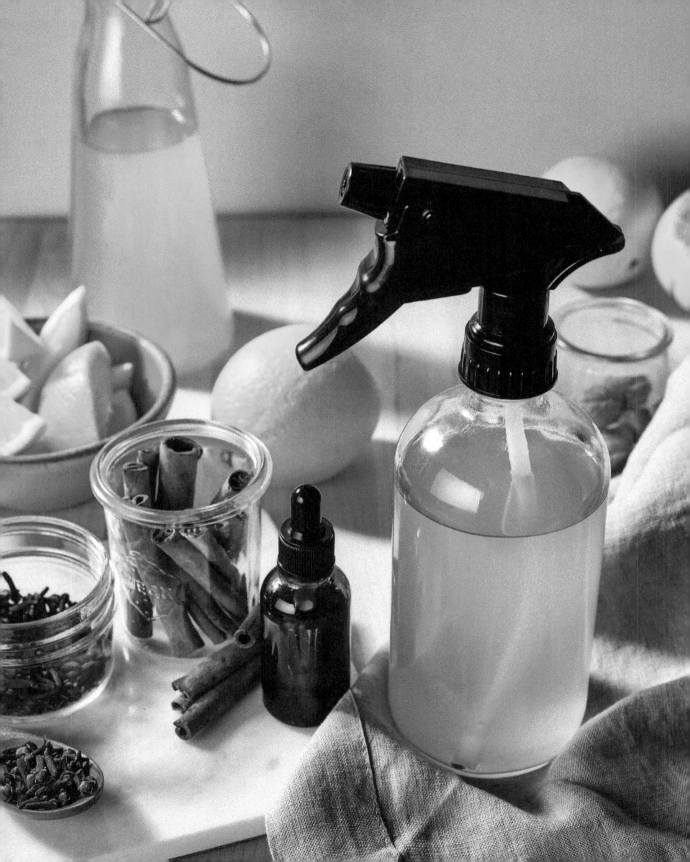

CHAPTER 4

Home

In this chapter, we will be delving into all the ways apple cider vinegar can be an effective part of cleaning and disinfecting your home. Apple cider vinegar contains properties that help remove bacteria and dirt buildup, kill bad odors, and disinfect. From all-purpose cleaners to wood polisher and weed killer, these amazing recipes for your home cover it all.

Cleansers

This section provides you with natural, effective recipes that will have your home sparkling from top to bottom without exposing your family and pets to unsafe chemicals.

FEATURED RECIPES: All-Purpose Citrus Kitchen Cleaner (114), Cinnamon-Clove Germs-Be-Gone Cleaning Spray (115), Mildew-Busting Rinse (116), Mold Treatment (117), Scorched Pans Stain Remover (118), Lemon-Lavender Refrigerator Cleaner (119), Cinnamon-Clove Coffee Maker Cleaner (120), Citrus Dishwasher Cleaner (121), Drain-Buster Solution (122), Simple Toilet Cleaner (123), Showerhead Unclogging Solution (124), Eucalyptus Washing Machine Refresher (125), Lemongrass Window and Mirror Cleaner (126), Tea Tree Phone Sanitizer (127), Simple Candle Wax Remover (128), Silver Cleaner (129), and Lemon Wood Polish Refresher (130).

ALL-PURPOSE CITRUS KITCHEN CLEANER

YIELD: 16 OUNCES | PREP TIME: 2 MINUTES

RECOMMENDED STORAGE: Store in a glass spray bottle.

This spray is my go-to cleaner at home. It has a refreshing, burst-of-citrus scent and is safe to use on kitchen counters and appliances. You can keep it under your sink and use it daily.

1 cup apple cider vinegar

1 cup water

2 tablespoons witch hazel

1 teaspoon liquid castile soap

10 drops lemongrass essential oil

10 drops grapefruit essential oil

1. Put the apple cider vinegar, water, witch hazel, castile soap, lemongrass essential oil, and grapefruit essential oil in a spray bottle. Shake well to combine.

2. Spray on kitchen counters and appliances and wipe with a paper towel or dishcloth.

CINNAMON-CLOVE GERMS-BE-GONE CLEANING SPRAY

YIELD: 16 OUNCES | PREP TIME: 2 MINUTES

RECOMMENDED STORAGE: Store in a glass spray bottle.

Studies have shown that clove possesses antimicrobial effects against bacteria. When combined with citrus, it has even more germ-, bacteria-, and mold-killing benefits. Cinnamon helps purify the surrounding air and provides an amazing smell in combination with the clove. This spray can be used all over the house from carpets to counters and tile surface areas.

1 cup apple cider vinegar

1 cup water

30 drops clove essential oil

20 drops cinnamon essential oil

15 drops lemon essential oil

1. Put the apple cider vinegar, water, clove essential oil, cinnamon essential oil, and lemon essential oil in a spray bottle. Shake well to combine.

2. Spray on surfaces and wait about 5 to 15 minutes before wiping the area clean. This allows the vinegar and oils to do their work.

3. Wipe the area with a paper towel or dishcloth.

MILDEW-BUSTING RINSE

YIELD: 16 OUNCES | PREP TIME: 2 MINUTES

RECOMMENDED STORAGE: Store in a glass spray bottle.

Inhaling or touching mildew can cause a variety of health problems, including allergies, cough, congestion, and bloody noses. This rinsing treatment provides a safe way to get rid of mildew in your home without using a chemical spray.

2 cups apple cider vinegar

15 drops oregano essential oil

15 drops thyme essential oil

1. Put the apple cider vinegar, oregano essential oil, and thyme essential oil in a spray bottle. Shake well to combine.

2. Spray on mildewy surfaces, scrub with a brush, and rinse.

3. Dry the area completely with a paper towel or dishcloth.

USAGE TIP: Use this rinse only on nonporous surfaces such as tile. Do not spray on wood.

MOLD TREATMENT

YIELD: 1 TREATMENT | PREP TIME: 5 MINUTES

SPECIAL MATERIALS NEEDED: Small scrubbing brush or toothbrush

RECOMMENDED STORAGE: Store in two glass spray bottles.

Mold is not only inconvenient but can also lead to a range of health issues. One of the most common ways to eliminate mold is with bleach, which is toxic and unsafe for both humans and pets because it contains chemicals that cause damage to the nervous system, the respiratory system, and other organs. This three-step treatment process eliminates mold without toxins or negative health effects. The first step will kill about 80 percent of mold and prevent it from coming back. The second step will work to remove signs of mold, leaving you with a clean surface. The third step will remove any mold that may still be lingering.

1 cup apple cider vinegar

1 tablespoon cinnamon essential oil

1 tablespoon tea tree essential oil

1 cup warm water

3 tablespoons baking soda

1 cup hydrogen peroxide

1. Put the apple cider vinegar, cinnamon essential oil, and tea tree essential oil in the first spray bottle. Seal the bottle and shake the mixture well to combine. Spray thoroughly onto the mold and let sit for at least 40 minutes before wiping the area clean.

2. In the second spray bottle, combine the water and baking soda. Seal and shake the bottle until the baking soda is fully dissolved. Spray thoroughly onto the mold and let sit for at least 40 minutes before wiping the area clean.

3. Dip a small scrubbing brush (or toothbrush) into the cup of hydrogen peroxide and scrub the mold. Continue to rinse the brush with water and dip back into the peroxide until there are no signs of mold.

4. When you have finished, do a final wipe of the surface with a paper towel or dishcloth. It is important that the area is left completely dry.

HEALTH TIP: Mold forms in areas that are dark and damp, so after you remove it, open windows and turn on fans to circulate air for at least an hour.

SCORCHED PANS STAIN REMOVER

YIELD: 1 TREATMENT | PREP TIME: 1 MINUTE | COOK TIME: 10 MINUTES

RECOMMENDED STORAGE: Storage is not recommended.

How frustrating is it when you're cooking an amazing meal and you walk away from the stove for a few minutes and come back to a completely scorched pan? You know, the kind where you spend forever soaking and scrubbing it and still cannot completely get rid of all the brown spots. This stain remover works great for scorched pans and takes the frustration out of cleaning. It includes simple, nontoxic items you can find right in your kitchen cabinet.

½ cup apple cider vinegar

½ cup water

1 to 2 tablespoons baking soda

1. Pour the apple cider vinegar and water into the scorched pan and heat on high on the stove until boiling.

2. Allow the mixture to boil for 1 minute, then remove from heat and pour the mixture down the drain.

3. Sprinkle the baking soda evenly on the inside of the pan and use a scrubbing sponge or pad to scrub the pan until all scorch spots are gone.

4. Rinse the pan with water and dry.

LEMON-LAVENDER REFRIGERATOR CLEANER

YIELD: 12 OUNCES | PREP TIME: 2 MINUTES

RECOMMENDED STORAGE: Store in a glass spray bottle.

I often feel like my refrigerator is clean one minute and a mess the next. I'm still not sure how that happens, but I rely heavily on this solution to keep my refrigerator sparkly clean and smelling super fresh. I love the combination of lemon and lavender, and my refrigerator smells phenomenal when I open it.

1 cup hot water

½ cup apple cider vinegar

20 drops lemon essential oil

10 drops lavender essential oil

1. In a spray bottle, combine the water, apple cider vinegar, lemon essential oil, and lavender essential oil.

2. Shake well before each use. After removing all food and items from the refrigerator, spray all over the inside, making sure to get all the shelves, drawers, sides, top, and bottom.

3. Let the solution sit for 10 minutes, then wipe clean with a sponge or paper towels.

USAGE TIP: Dip a toothbrush in the solution to get it into hard-to-reach places.

CINNAMON-CLOVE COFFEE MAKER CLEANER

YIELD: 1 (72-OUNCE) APPLICATION | PREP TIME: 2 MINUTES

RECOMMENDED STORAGE: Storage is not recommended.

If you haven't been regularly cleaning your coffee maker, you are missing out. So much buildup occurs in coffee makers because of the thick grinds that seem to get stuck everywhere. This solution will break down the buildup and coffee particles, extend the life of your coffee maker, and best of all, make your coffee taste better.

6 cups water

3 cups apple cider vinegar

5 drops cinnamon essential oil

5 drops clove essential oil

1. Before beginning, make sure to dump out any leftover coffee from the pot and empty the filter compartment.

2. Fill the coffee pot with the water, apple cider vinegar, cinnamon essential oil, and clove essential oil. If your coffee pot is small, adjust the amounts while maintaining a 1:2 ratio of apple cider vinegar to water.

3. Pour the mixture into the opening where you would normally pour in water to make coffee.

4. Turn on the coffee maker and set to "brew."

5. Once the brewing is complete, let the solution sit for 10 to 15 minutes.

6. Discard the liquid and repeat the process with just water for 2 to 3 cycles to ensure that there is no remaining vinegar.

CITRUS DISHWASHER CLEANER

YIELD: 1 APPLICATION | PREP TIME: 2 MINUTES

RECOMMENDED STORAGE: Storage is not recommended.

Citrus makes everything feel so fresh, and it is very uplifting for the mood. And why not be extra happy in the kitchen? In addition to cleaning my kitchen with citrus-infused natural cleaners, such as the All-Purpose Citrus Kitchen Cleaner (page 114), I also love to clean my dishwasher with citrus. Not only does it remove soap, food, and bacteria buildup, but it also gives the dishwasher an amazing citrus scent. All that buildup actually makes the dishwasher less effective over time, so I like to run this cycle once a month to keep my dishwasher working its best.

1 cup apple cider vinegar

20 drops lemon essential oil

20 drops sweet orange essential oil

1. Place a dishwasher-safe mug in the dishwasher facing up on the top rack.

2. Pour the apple cider vinegar, lemon essential oil, and sweet orange essential oil into the mug.

3. Run your dishwasher on the hottest and longest cycle.

PREPARATION TIP: Before running the cycle, remove any food particles or buildup in the drain. This action will increase efficiency.

DRAIN-BUSTER SOLUTION

YIELD: 1 (12-OUNCE) APPLICATION | PREP TIME: 2 MINUTES

RECOMMENDED STORAGE: Storage is not recommended.

Unclogging your drain can get expensive. If you are constantly buying a solvent from the grocery store or having to call a plumber, it adds up. This is a great way to maintain a clear drain so that you can avoid future expenses. It is quick, easy, and cost-effective. As an added bonus, it helps eliminate sink odor.

1 cup apple cider vinegar

30 drops lemon essential oil

½ cup baking soda

1. In a cup, combine the apple cider vinegar and lemon essential oil.
2. Using a funnel, pour the baking soda down the drain.
3. Pour the apple cider vinegar mixture down the drain.
4. The combination of the baking soda and vinegar will foam up. When the foam subsides, turn on the hot water and flush the mixture for about 15 seconds.
5. If the drain is still clogged, repeat the process.
6. When you are finished, turn on the cold water and flush for another 15 seconds.

SIMPLE TOILET CLEANER

YIELD: 1 (4-OUNCE) APPLICATION | PREP TIME: 2 MINUTES

RECOMMENDED STORAGE: Storage is not recommended.

Nothing is worse than a dirty toilet bowl. I love when the bowl is sparkling clean and fresh smelling, but that just-cleaned bleach smell can be unpleasant. This simple recipe is inexpensive and nontoxic, and it will leave a natural fresh scent long after you are done cleaning.

½ cup apple cider vinegar

20 drops lemon essential oil

20 drops sweet orange essential oil

1. Pour the apple cider vinegar into your toilet bowl and scrub the inside of the bowl with a toilet brush.

2. Let the mixture sit in the bowl for at least 30 minutes. (You can also leave it in overnight.)

3. Scrub the inside of the bowl again until it is clean, then flush the mixture.

4. Add the essential oils to the fresh toilet bowl water.

5. Use the toilet brush to mix the oils in the water and then scrub the sides of the bowl.

6. Let sit at least 30 minutes and flush when finished.

SHOWERHEAD UNCLOGGING SOLUTION

YIELD: 1 (16-OUNCE) APPLICATION | PREP TIME: 2 MINUTES

RECOMMENDED STORAGE: Storage is not recommended.

I love this simple vinegar hack. Mold, mildew, and bacteria can build up in the showerhead because of the constant moisture. When you turn the shower on, that buildup gets released into the air for you to breathe. This solution is a great reboot to clean your showerhead naturally so that it is safe and works more efficiently.

2 cups apple cider vinegar

30 drops lemon essential oil

1. Use a wet cloth to wipe your showerhead clean and remove extra debris and buildup.
2. Pour the apple cider vinegar and lemon essential oil into a plastic bag and pull the bag up over the showerhead, making sure the holes where the water comes out are fully immersed in the solution.
3. Using a twist tie or string, tie the bag tight so that the showerhead stays immersed.
4. Allow the showerhead to soak in the solution for at least one hour.
5. When finished, remove the bag and wipe the showerhead clean with a paper towel or dishcloth.

EUCALYPTUS WASHING MACHINE REFRESHER

YIELD: 1 APPLICATION | PREP TIME: 1 MINUTE

RECOMMENDED STORAGE: Storage is not recommended.

It may seem silly that a machine that cleans clothes also needs cleaning, but it does. Bacteria, mold, and mildew can build up in your machine over time. Cleaning your washing machine makes a huge difference in the way it functions. Giving it a deep cleaning allows your clothes to come out smelling even better.

NOTE: If your washing machine is still under warranty, check the conditions to make sure that using anything other than chlorinated bleach will not void your warranty.

4 cups *or* ¾ cup apple cider vinegar

15 drops eucalyptus essential oil

1. Set your washing machine to the longest cycle and the hottest temperature. (If this is not an option, select "whites.")

2. **For top-loaders:** Once hot water is running, add 4 cups of apple cider vinegar to the water. Let it run for 5 to 10 minutes. Then stop the cycle and let the vinegar and water sit for 1 hour. Use this time to scrub hard-to-reach spots internally and externally on the machine. Dip a rag into the vinegar and water, wring it out, and scrub areas such as the bleach compartment and knobs. After an hour, close the lid and finish the washing cycle.

   For front-loaders: Pour ¾ cup of apple cider vinegar into the bleach dispenser until it is filled to its maximum level. Run the washing cycle until it is completed.

3. For both types of machines, when the first washing cycle is complete, set the machine to the longest cycle and hottest temperature again. Add the eucalyptus essential oil in the same manner and let the cycle run its course.

LEMONGRASS WINDOW AND MIRROR CLEANER

YIELD: 16 OUNCES | PREP TIME: 2 MINUTES

RECOMMENDED STORAGE: Store in a glass spray bottle.

Want that streak-free look to your windows and mirrors? Using apple cider vinegar achieves this. Not only does it clean without the streaks, but it also breaks down the film and bacteria that accumulate on glass surfaces. This cleaner is a safe, nontoxic alternative to traditional cleaners, so you can feel good about spraying it around kids and pets.

1 cup apple cider vinegar

1 cup water

30 drops lemongrass essential oil

1. In a spray bottle, combine the apple cider vinegar, water, and lemongrass essential oil.
2. Shake well before each use. Spray on glass surfaces and wipe with a sponge or cloth from the top down.

USAGE TIP: Clean glass surfaces only when sunlight is not directly on them, because the heat will cause surfaces to dry too fast and they will streak.

TEA TREE PHONE SANITIZER

YIELD: 5 OUNCES | PREP TIME: 2 MINUTES

RECOMMENDED STORAGE: Store in a glass spray bottle.

Our phones are covered with bacteria. In fact, they are likely one of the dirtiest things we touch all day. Think about all the surfaces a phone comes in contact with, including other people's hands. That is why regularly cleaning your phone is extremely important. This recipe is a perfect, safe, nontoxic solution for cleaning your phone that won't leave you with breakouts when your phone has been up to your ear.

½ cup water

1 tablespoon apple cider vinegar

1 tablespoon witch hazel

10 drops tea tree essential oil

1. In a small spray bottle, combine the water, apple cider vinegar, witch hazel, and tea tree essential oil.

2. Shake well, spray 2 to 4 pumps onto a microfiber cloth, and wipe your phone clean. Never spray directly onto your phone.

SIMPLE CANDLE WAX REMOVER

YIELD: 1 (4-OUNCE) APPLICATION | PREP TIME: 2 MINUTES

SPECIAL MATERIALS NEEDED: Hair dryer

RECOMMENDED STORAGE: Storage is not recommended.

At one point or another, we have probably all had to remove wax that dripped, whether a candle was accidentally knocked over or we forgot to put a tray underneath it to catch the drips. This remedy works great for removing candle wax from wood surfaces such as coffee tables, desks, or side tables. Keep in mind, this solution will *not* remove candle wax from carpet.

¼ cup apple cider vinegar

¼ cup water (plus more for a final rinse)

1. Heat the candle wax with a hair dryer on high heat to soften. Gently blot up as much wax as you can with a paper towel.
2. In a glass bowl, combine the apple cider vinegar and water. Dip one side of a dishcloth into the mixture, wring it out, and wipe the wax until the surface is clean.
3. When all the wax is gone, dip the other side of the dishcloth in just water and wipe the surface clean to make sure there is no vinegar residue.
4. Dry the area completely.

SILVER CLEANER

YIELD: 1 (2-OUNCE) APPLICATION | PREP TIME: 1 MINUTE

RECOMMENDED STORAGE: Storage is not recommended.

This cleaning solution is fantastic for silver jewelry. I regularly soak my silver earrings in it to give them a good cleaning. It also works really well on stainless steel and chrome items such as sinks, faucets, and stainless steel appliances. It gives everything a brand-new shiny look and kills surface bacteria.

¼ cup apple cider vinegar

10 drops lime essential oil

1. Put the silver you want to clean in a small bowl.
2. Add the apple cider vinegar and lime essential oil and give it a light swirl with your fingers to combine.
3. Let the silver sit in the mixture for 5 to 10 minutes.
4. Remove the silver, rinse with cold water, and dry with a paper towel or microfiber towel.

> **USAGE TIP:** For stainless steel and chrome surfaces, you can dip a rag in the solution and wipe to clean.

LEMON WOOD POLISH REFRESHER

YIELD: 10 OUNCES | PREP TIME: 2 MINUTES

RECOMMENDED STORAGE: Store in a glass spray bottle.

This refresher gives your wood a new, bright look while also removing water marks and stains. It is a great all-purpose solution for the wood furniture around your home. Olive oil creates shine by moisturizing the wood and also protects it. Apple cider vinegar breaks down any grimy buildup on the surface. Lemon juice disinfects while adding a pleasant scent to the cleaner.

1 cup olive oil

¼ cup apple cider vinegar

1 tablespoon freshly squeezed lemon juice

20 drops lemongrass essential oil

1. Put the olive oil, apple cider vinegar, lemon juice, and lemongrass essential oil in a spray bottle. Shake to combine.

2. Spray the mixture onto wood surfaces and rub with a microfiber cloth.

Deodorizers

When your home is not smelling as fresh as it could, these easy recipes will reinvigorate your space, as well as your clothing, shoes, couches, and carpets. Changing the scents around you can also lift your spirits and provide you with the energy you need to accomplish more throughout the day.

FEATURED RECIPES: Lavender-Peppermint Clothes Disinfectant Spray (132), Stinky Shoe Disinfectant Spray (133), Citrus Couch Sanitizer (134), Rosemary-and-Grapefruit-Infused Carpet Refresher (135), Peppermint-Eucalyptus Deodorizing Spray (136), and Holiday Spice Room Refresher (137).

LAVENDER-PEPPERMINT CLOTHES DISINFECTANT SPRAY

YIELD: 12 OUNCES | PREP TIME: 2 MINUTES

RECOMMENDED STORAGE: Store in a glass spray bottle.

I love using apple cider vinegar as a simple hack for keeping laundry fresh and free of odors. It contains acetic acid, which works to soften and brighten fabrics and kill odors when it comes to laundry. It can also help reduce lint and pet hair, banish mildew smells, keep dark clothing dark, and get rid of underarm odor. This spray is a great replacement for fabric softener, which contains toxic chemicals and is a known pore clogger that can lead to acne breakouts.

1 cup water

½ cup apple cider vinegar

15 drops lavender essential oil

10 drops peppermint essential oil

1. Put the water, apple cider vinegar, lavender essential oil, and peppermint essential oil in a small bottle.

2. Shake well before each use and hold the bottle about 2 feet from the clothes you are spraying. You want to spray a light mist, not get the clothes wet.

USAGE TIP: I recommend using this treatment for T-shirts, workout clothes, and clothing made of cotton or denim. If you are going to use it on a high-quality fabric item, first test a patch on the inside of the clothing, near a bottom hemline.

STINKY SHOE DISINFECTANT SPRAY

YIELD: 16 OUNCES | PREP TIME: 2 MINUTES

RECOMMENDED STORAGE: Store in a glass spray bottle.

Stinky shoes lead to stinky feet! After you spend an entire day in your shoes or your kiddos come home from playing outside, stinky shoes can be hard to avoid. The solution is this disinfectant spray. You can use it daily or when you feel like your shoes could use a little refresh. When used regularly, it will neutralize foot odor, but don't worry, your feet won't smell like apple cider vinegar. Once the spray dries, the vinegar scent disappears.

1 cup water

½ cup apple cider vinegar

½ cup witch hazel

30 drops peppermint essential oil

30 drops tea tree essential oil

1. In a spray bottle combine the water, apple cider vinegar, witch hazel, peppermint essential oil, and tea tree essential oil.

2. Shake well before each use and mist on the inside and outside of shoes. You can wipe the outside with a towel or cloth but let the inside air-dry.

USAGE TIP: This disinfectant spray can also be used on stinky sports equipment. It is a huge helper that keeps your car, home, and laundry room smelling fresh.

CITRUS COUCH SANITIZER

YIELD: 16 OUNCES | PREP TIME: 2 MINUTES

RECOMMENDED STORAGE: Store in a glass spray bottle.

Lime and grapefruit essential oils provide a great uplifting scent, making this sanitizer a great after-spray for when you need to give your couch a refresh. I also love spraying it before someone sleeps on the couch because it leaves a welcoming citrus smell.

1 cup apple cider vinegar

1 cup water

30 drops lime essential oil

30 drops grapefruit essential oil

1. In a spray bottle as elsewhere combine the apple cider vinegar, water, lime essential oil, and grapefruit essential oil.

2. Shake well before each use and spray at least 2 feet away from the couch. You want to mist the couch, not get it wet.

ROSEMARY-AND-GRAPEFRUIT-INFUSED CARPET REFRESHER

YIELD: 16 OUNCES | PREP TIME: 5 MINUTES | INFUSION TIME: 10 TO 14 DAYS

RECOMMENDED STORAGE: Store in a 16-ounce (or larger) glass jar with lid and a glass spray bottle.

I love this recipe because the combination of grapefruit and rosemary makes for such a refreshing scent. This spray is great to use after vacuuming or cleaning the carpets to add antibacterial and antifungal benefits and make the room smell super clean. Because of the infusion of citrus and herbs, it does not have a strong vinegar smell.

1 grapefruit, peel only

3 to 5 rosemary sprigs

15 drops grapefruit essential oil

2 cups apple cider vinegar

Water

1. Put the grapefruit peel, rosemary sprigs, and grapefruit essential oil in a large glass jar.

2. Pour the apple cider vinegar into the jar, covering the grapefruit peel and rosemary. (If the amount doesn't cover, you can add more apple cider vinegar.) Seal the jar and shake until the mixture is well combined.

3. Let the mixture sit to infuse for 10 to 14 days.

4. Strain out the solids and put the infused vinegar back in the jar.

5. Add equal parts water and the infused vinegar to a spray bottle. Seal the bottle and shake to combine.

6. Store the leftover infused vinegar in the sealed jar and use it to refill the spray bottle as you run out, adding equal parts water.

7. Shake well before each use and spray the carpet from about 2 feet away.

VARIATION TIP: To make the grapefruit and rosemary scent even stronger, add additional drops of grapefruit essential oil and several drops of rosemary essential oil to the spray bottle after preparing the mixture.

PEPPERMINT-EUCALYPTUS DEODORIZING SPRAY

YIELD: 10 OUNCES | PREP TIME: 2 MINUTES

RECOMMENDED STORAGE: Store in a glass spray bottle.

This spray can be used to refresh clothes, shoes, your car, or anything that has a stinky smell you need to get rid of. Both peppermint and eucalyptus have strong scents that cancel out unpleasant odors. I keep a small container of this spray in my car to use as needed.

1 cup water

¼ cup apple cider vinegar

10 to 15 drops peppermint essential oil

7 drops eucalyptus essential oil

1. Put the water, apple cider vinegar, peppermint essential oil, and eucalyptus essential oil in a spray bottle. Shake well to combine.
2. Shake well before each use and hold the bottle about 12 inches from the item you are spraying.

HOLIDAY SPICE ROOM REFRESHER

YIELD: 12 OUNCES | PREP TIME: 2 MINUTES

RECOMMENDED STORAGE: Store in a glass spray bottle.

I love the scents around the holidays. Pine, cinnamon, cloves . . . it all smells so cozy. One of my favorite things to do is to spray this room refresher around the house so that it smells like the holidays all the time. This spray has a punch of cinnamon spice along with some other amazing holiday scents to get you in the spirit. It is also a great alternative to the many toxic sprays known for their seasonal aromas.

1 cup water

½ cup apple cider vinegar

30 drops cinnamon essential oil

15 drops sweet orange essential oil

10 drops nutmeg essential oil

10 drops clove essential oil

1. In a spray bottle, combine the water, apple cider vinegar, cinnamon essential oil, sweet orange essential oil, nutmeg essential oil, and clove essential oil.

2. Shake well before each use and spray wherever you would like around your home.

Insects, Pets, and Weeds

Warmer weather can bring some pesky invaders with it. This section will cover recipes to eliminate insects in your home, skin irritation for dogs, and weeds in your garden. Because these recipes are all natural, you won't have to worry about contaminating your food or harming pets or plants with dangerous chemicals.

FEATURED RECIPES: Kitchen-Safe Insect Spray (page 139), Soothing Itch Spray for Dogs (page 140), Natural Weed Killer (page 141).

KITCHEN-SAFE INSECT SPRAY

YIELD: 10 OUNCES | PREP TIME: 2 MINUTES

RECOMMENDED STORAGE: Store in a glass spray bottle.

Dealing with insects in the kitchen can be difficult. Chemical repellents have the potential to get into food and cause health problems if ingested. This spray is a safe alternative for getting rid of insects, and it would still be safe if any lingering spray were to come in contact with food. Tea tree and peppermint essential oils are powerful killers of both spiders and ants, while lemongrass essential oil repels and kills ticks, chiggers, fleas, and flies.

1 cup grain alcohol
(vodka will work)

¼ cup apple cider vinegar

3 teaspoons olive oil

20 drops tea tree essential oil

20 drops peppermint
essential oil

20 drops lemongrass
essential oil

1. Put the alcohol, apple cider vinegar, olive oil, tea tree essential oil, peppermint essential oil, and lemongrass essential oil in a spray bottle. Shake well to combine.

2. Several times a day, spray the infested areas of your home until the insects are gone.

SOOTHING ITCH
SPRAY FOR DOGS

YIELD: 8 OUNCES | PREP TIME: 2 MINUTES

RECOMMENDED STORAGE: Store in a glass spray bottle in the refrigerator for up to 1 year.

When your dog is constantly scratching, it can be super uncomfortable for them. This spray is the perfect relief, not only to ease itchy, irritated skin, but also to prevent future dry skin. The chamomile tea creates a soothing effect for your dog's irritated skin while the apple cider vinegar serves as an antiseptic and antifungal that provides additional relief. Vitamin E oil is known to provide allergy relief for dogs as well as help with dandruff and dry skin.

¾ cup brewed and cooled chamomile tea

¼ cup apple cider vinegar

1 tablespoon Vitamin E oil

1. In the spray bottle, combine chamomile tea, apple cider vinegar, and Vitamin E oil. Seal the bottle and shake the mixture well to combine.

2. Spray on dog's skin as needed, avoiding face area, open wounds, and raw skin.

NATURAL WEED KILLER

YIELD: 26 OUNCES | PREP TIME: 2 MINUTES

RECOMMENDED STORAGE: Store in a glass spray bottle.

Most weed killers contain toxic chemicals that can be harmful not only to people but also to pets. Toxic weed killers have been linked to cancer, kidney and liver damage, and endocrine disruption. A natural solution is safer because you do not have to worry about any toxicity poisoning while you are gardening, or while your pets or children are playing in the yard.

3 cups apple cider vinegar

½ cup salt

¼ cup orange (or any citrus) essential oil

½ tablespoon liquid dish soap

1. Put the apple cider vinegar, salt, orange essential oil, and liquid dish soap in a large spray bottle.

2. Seal the bottle and give it a light shake. You want to combine everything but not create too many bubbles.

3. Spray directly on the weeds and roots, making sure to avoid the plants you want to keep alive.

> USAGE TIP: Time of day and weather conditions are very important for best results. Apply when there is direct sunlight, preferably during the hottest part of the day. The weeds should be dry, so if it has rained recently and weeds are still wet or damp, don't apply.

Conversion Tables

VOLUME EQUIVALENTS (LIQUID)

US STANDARD	US STANDARD (OUNCES)	METRIC (APPROXIMATE)
2 tablespoons	1 fl. oz.	30 mL
¼ cup	2 fl. oz.	60 mL
½ cup	4 fl. oz.	120 mL
1 cup	8 fl. oz.	240 mL
1½ cups	12 fl. oz.	355 mL
2 cups or 1 pint	16 fl. oz.	475 mL
4 cups or 1 quart	32 fl. oz.	1 L
1 gallon	128 fl. oz.	4 L

OVEN TEMPERATURES

FAHRENHEIT (F)	CELSIUS (C) (APPROXIMATE)
250°F	120°C
300°F	150°C
325°F	165°C
350°F	180°C
375°F	190°C
400°F	200°C
425°F	220°C
450°F	230°C

VOLUME EQUIVALENTS (DRY)

US STANDARD	METRIC (APPROXIMATE)
⅛ teaspoon	0.5 mL
¼ teaspoon	1 mL
½ teaspoon	2 mL
¾ teaspoon	4 mL
1 teaspoon	5 mL
1 tablespoon	15 mL
¼ cup	59 mL
⅓ cup	79 mL
½ cup	118 mL
⅔ cup	156 mL
¾ cup	177 mL
1 cup	235 mL
2 cups or 1 pint	475 mL
3 cups	700 mL
4 cups or 1 quart	1 L

WEIGHT EQUIVALENTS

US STANDARD	METRIC (APPROXIMATE)
½ ounce	15 g
1 ounce	30 g
2 ounces	60 g
4 ounces	115 g
8 ounces	225 g
12 ounces	340 g
16 ounces or 1 pound	455 g

Resources

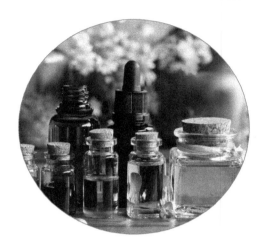

High-Quality Essential Oils

DOTERRA
doterra.com/US/en/

YOUNG LIVING
youngliving.com/en_US/

Raw, Unfiltered Apple Cider Vinegar

BRAGG
bragg.com/products/bragg-organic-apple-cider-vinegar.html

COMPLETE NATURAL PRODUCTS
completenaturalproducts.com/apple-cider-vinegar-unfiltered-kosher
-usda-organic-with-the-mother

DYNAMIC HEALTH

dynamichealth.com/apple-cider-vinegar-w-mother-certified-organic-1.html

THRIVE MARKET

thrivemarket.com/p/thrive-market-organic-apple-cider-vinegar

High-Quality Teas

NUMI ORGANIC TEA

numitea.com

TRADITIONAL MEDICINALS

traditionalmedicinals.com

STASH TEA COMPANY

stashtea.com

YOGI

yogiproducts.com

High-Quality Medicinal Mushroom Powders

FOUR SIGMATIC

us.foursigmatic.com

OM MUSHROOM SUPERFOOD

ommushrooms.com

Reusable Straws

finalstraw.com

simplystraws.com

References

Budak, Nilgün H., Elif Aykin, Atif C. Seydim, Annel K. Greene, and Zeynep B. Guzel-Seydim. "Functional Properties of Vinegar." *Journal of Food Science* 74, no. 5 (May 2014): R757–R764. doi: 10.1111/1750-3841.12434. https://onlinelibrary .wiley.com/doi/full/10.1111/1750-3841.12434.

Hellmiss, Margot. *Natural Healing with Apple Cider Vinegar.* New York: Sterling Publishing, 1996.

Johnston, Carol S., and Cindy A. Gaas. "Vinegar: Medicinal Uses and Antiglycemic Effect." *Medscape General Medicine* 8, no. 2 (2006): 6. Published online May 2006. https://www.ncbi.nlm.nih.gov/pmc/articles/PMC1785201

Jones, Bridget. *Vinegar and Oil.* London: Anness Publishing, Lorenz Books, 2010.

Kondo, S., K. Tayama, Y. Tsukamoto, K. Ikeda, and Y. Yamori. "Antihypertensive Effects of Acetic Acid and Vinegar on Spontaneously Hypertensive Rats." *Bioscience, Biotechnology, and Biochemistry.* (2001): 65:02690–2694. https://www.ncbi.nlm.nih.gov/pubmed/11826965.

Liljeberg, Helena, and I. Björck. "Delayed Gastric Emptying Rate May Explain Improved Glycemia in Healthy Subjects to a Starchy Meal with Added Vinegar." *European Journal of Clinical Nutrition* 64 (1998):886–893. https://www.ncbi.nlm.nih.gov/pubmed/9630389.

"Literature Review Health Benefits Apple Cider Vinegar, Acidic Fermented Apple Peel and Grape Extracts." Australian Functional Nutraceutical, Botanical Innovations https://botanicalinnovations.com.au/wp-content/uploads/2017/03 /literature-review-health-benefits-apple-cider-vinegar-fermented-grape -apple-extracts1.pdf.

Mercola, Joseph MD. "What the Research Really Says About Apple Cider Vinegar." Mercola.com. June 2, 2009. https://articles.mercola.com/sites/articles/archive/2009/06/02/apple-cider-vinegar-hype.aspx.

Rund, C. R. "Nonconventional Topical Therapies for Wound Care." *Ostomy Wound Management*. (1996): 42:22–24. https://www.ncbi.nlm.nih.gov/pubmed/8717010.

Rutala, William A., Susan L. Barbee, Newman C. Aguiar, Mark D. Sobsey, and David J. Weber. "Antimicrobial Activity of Home Disinfectants and Natural Products Against Potential Human Pathogens." *Infection Control and Hospital Epidemiology*. (2000): 21:33–38. https://www.ncbi.nlm.nih.gov/pubmed/10656352.

Takano-Lee M, Edman JD, Mullens BA, Clark JM. "Home Remedies to Control Head Lice: Assessment of Home Remedies to Control the Human Head Louse, Pediculus Humanus Capitis (Anoplura: Pediculidae)." *Journal of Pediatric Nursing*. (2004):19:393–398. https://www.ncbi.nlm.nih.gov/pubmed/15637580.

Vinegars and Acetic Acid Bacteria. International Symposium, May, 2005; Available at: http://www.vinegars2005.com/images/Vin_2005_book.pdf. Accessed March 9, 2006.

Index

About the Author

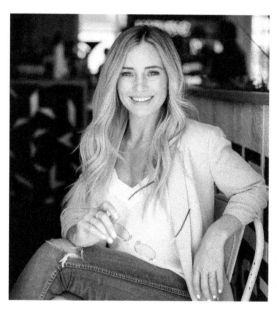

© Hannah Claire Photography

KAYLEIGH CHRISTINA CLARK, the cofounder of CLEARstem Skincare, is a holistic nutritionist and certified health coach with a keen understanding of the ingredients we put in our bodies for better or worse. She has struggled with leaky gut, ovarian cysts, a breast tumor, and severe cystic acne. She developed celiac disease in her mid-twenties and tried in vain to find relief. She ultimately found healing by taking a whole-body approach to wellness, including changing the foods she was putting into her body and the products she was using topically. Clark is also the cohost of the "Balancing Your Hustle" podcast on iTunes and GooglePlay, which focuses on balancing career, passions, and wellness.

CPSIA information can be obtained
at www.ICGtesting.com
Printed in the USA
BVHW052143281019
562301BV00002B/47/P